Inconceivable

A MEMOIR

Inconceivable

A MEMOIR

Super Sperm Donors, Off-the-Grid Insemination, and Unconventional Family Planning

Valerie Bauman

UNION
SQUARE
& CO.

NEW YORK

UNION SQUARE & CO.

NEW YORK

ISBN 978-1-4549-5143-8
ISBN 978-1-4549-5144-5 (e-book)

Library of Congress Control Number: 2023048598
Library of Congress Cataloging-in-Publication Data is available upon request.

For information about custom editions, special sales, and premium purchases,
please contact specialsales@unionsquareandco.com.

Printed in the United States of America

2   4   6   8   10   9   7   5   3   1

unionsquareandco.com

Cover design by Elizabeth Mihaltse Lindy
Cover images by Shutterstock.com: Arcady (sperm); Ron Dale (egg)
Interior design by Rich Hazelton

For Luna, who showed me new depths of love in such a short time.
May we meet again.

And for Mom, for never—not once—making me doubt your love was
unconditional. But, seriously, please don't read this book.
No need to test that theory.

"Having a child is to show an absolute accord with mankind. If I have a child, it's as though I'm saying: I was born and have tasted life and declare it so good that it merits being duplicated."

—Milan Kundera
Farewell Waltz

Contents

Preface

IT WAS ONE OF THOSE impossibly long days during the first summer of the COVID-19 pandemic in Washington, D.C.

I took a deep drag on my cigarette before stubbing it out and looking around at the backyard, a decrepit, brick-laden private paradise covered in overgrown ivy, lush flowers, and plants that I tended to myself. It was June and I could smell the mosquito repellent as it evaporated off my skin. I was surrounded by vivid splashes of pink, orange, yellow, and purple, having planted a mix of snapdragons, pansies, black-eyed Susans, dianthus, and other flowers, two months prior.

Nestled in the heart of Capitol Hill, my apartment had the rare luxury of a massive outdoor space. I got lucky finding my one-bedroom when I arrived from Brooklyn the year before.

Even better than the surroundings? The neighbors. They made living through a pandemic a little bit easier. Avery, a nonbinary friend with vivid pink hair who lived in an apartment kitty-corner to mine, peered at me from across the patio furniture.

"What? What are you thinking about?" Avery asked, putting out a cigarette.

"I think I want to have a baby," I said, surprising myself by letting the words slip out loud before taking a sip of whiskey.

"Oh! You totally should!" Avery loved babies.

I started rolling us a fresh joint as I contemplated the idea. I was a thirty-eight-year-old journalist who had spent the past decade and a half crisscrossing the country for my career, working fifty to sixty hours a week. I had a nearly pack-a-day habit and was a regular at the dive bar around the corner.

My apartment was 650 square feet and littered with half-empty seltzer cans, small piles of unopened mail, and a few take-out containers. I don't think I could have done a more blatant impression of the whiskey-swigging, workaholic reporter stereotype if I tried. But it wasn't an act. My lifestyle, especially during the pandemic, was less Lois Lane and more Jimmy Breslin (before he quit drinking).

I was a bit of a disaster.

But that's not the whole story. I had also rebounded from being a high school dropout and managed to turn my love of words into a successful journalism career. I had gone to community college and a small state school, yet I was scrappy enough to get to work alongside some of the most talented people in the business—most of whom seemed to come from Ivy League backgrounds. I had a reputation for bringing passion and a fierce work ethic to all that I did, which helped me get promoted to senior investigative reporter—my dream job—in the middle of a pandemic. Career-wise, I'd pretty much grown up to be exactly who I always hoped to be.

Beyond that, I tried to be a good friend who conscientiously tended to those relationships across decades and time zones, dropping everything to fly cross-country when someone I loved was in need. I was also a big sister who learned a lot from helping my mom care for my three little brothers.

I was always a nurturer; I just didn't nurture myself. On some level, I didn't think I deserved love—romantic or otherwise. Not that I hadn't tried. I felt ready to settle down and have kids around the age of twenty-five or twenty-six. I had several long-term relationships in my twenties and thirties, spanning one to six years. I was always up front with men about my desire to get married and have multiple children; several men said they wanted that, too, with me. Every time, years would pass, and they still weren't ready.

The men I connected with in my generation were often in some Peter Pan state of emotional cryogenics that made them want to have the freedom to date and sleep with as many people as possible without ever making a commitment. Polyamory and ethical non-monogamy were now a thing—which, cool. Just not for me. Now I was single and thirty-eight years old, and men my age were looking to have children with women in their twenties and early thirties. Meanwhile, I was still hitting snooze on my biological clock. Time was running out to pursue the one thing

I've always known I wanted: to be a mom. And maybe, perhaps, something that big could actually be the catalyst for me to sort my life out.

Even if I had to do it alone.

I shivered in spite of the summer heat.

"Nah," I told Avery. "I could never do it on my own."

But the idea wouldn't leave me. It was a whisper, tickling the back of my skull as I tried to fall asleep for several nights in a row. Finally, a few days later, I was watering the flowers in the same garden, observing how beautifully they responded to my care and attention. And I had an epiphany: I *could* do it. I, Valerie Bauman, could have a baby on my own. No one could prevent me from pursuing this. No one was going to give me permission, either. It was entirely my decision—I'm still not clear on why that was such a jarring realization. But it was. And from that moment, I knew I was going to go through with it.

Making the decision was simple. But I never could have anticipated where this choice would take me, or the lengths I would go to become a parent on my own terms. Nothing about finding a sperm donor, or the journey to motherhood, came easy for me.

Chapter One
Chasing Babies

THEY INSEMINATE THEMSELVES IN CARS, public restrooms, and cheap motel rooms. They pray over urine-drenched sticks, guzzle supplements by the dozen, and sometimes have unprotected sex with men they've only just met on the internet, Facebook groups, or dating-like apps—whatever it takes to make their baby dreams come true.

What could possibly drive a woman out of the cool, clinical embrace of the health-care industry for one of the biggest medical decisions of her life? For some it's the insurmountable costs imposed by the reproductive industry, or discrimination, or a lack of insurance coverage. Others just want to know the person who will help create their child.

I am one of those women. Like most, I started out scrolling through the sperm bank websites, analyzing donor profiles and squinting at their baby pictures. I even made a color-coded spreadsheet (green for positive attributes, red for negative, and yellow for things that gave me pause). But like many women, I soon realized that sperm banks weren't the answer, not for me. I wanted to know the person who would help me create my child, to be able to give my kid answers and insights into where they came from.

This is a story of spitting in the face of virtually every cultural taboo around family, fertility, and procreation for the sake of making motherhood a reality.

IN JULY 2020, SHORTLY AFTER my revelation that I could become a mother on my own terms, I sat curled up on the couch, computer in my lap, compulsively scrolling through various sperm bank websites. Over several days I built the spreadsheet entitled "Babies." I added nineteen columns that listed the characteristics I could find on each donor using whatever details the banks provided for free—and what I could glean from photos.

Some of the characteristics were physical: height, weight, build. Eye color and hair color are always listed, but some banks even provide details on the donor's hair texture and thickness. Race and ethnicity were also included. I added the category of "Lips," largely based on what I could tell from available photos—purely because I'm a fan of full lips and got a little carried away with the spreadsheet.

Other categories were more practical, including sperm motility and price, and whether the donor had any reported pregnancies or children of his own. Sometimes the gender of the donor's children was listed, which was helpful, I suppose, for those who had a gender preference. I was more interested in their job and education. I was surprised by some of the information that was available—things I hadn't thought to ask about, like allergies or shoe size. I was tickled by the banks that listed which famous actor the donor most resembled (according to the discerning opinions of sperm bank staff).

These weren't necessarily the things I cared about most. But it's all I could learn from what the banks provided for free. You had to pay more for adult photos on most sites, as well as for a detailed family history and other information on the individual donor. At California Cryobank, which advertises itself as the largest sperm bank in the world, for the bargain price of $145, you get ninety days of access to seeing adult and additional childhood photos of donors, as well as an extended donor profile and a keepsake of some kind from the donor—such as a poem, original song composition, or something else that allows him to express himself. If you shell out $250, you get all of that—for ninety days only—and a detailed report on his facial features, an extensive temperament/personality test result, and an audio recording of the donor's voice that can be saved for the child to hear later.

My cat, Ruby, watched—heartless in her indifference—as I tossed my computer on the couch and paced around my tiny living room contemplating the options. I ran through the donors in my head, occasionally pausing to review my spreadsheet as I weighed each one. It was overwhelming, because one moment I'd be so enamored with a particular donor (all of whom had fake names assigned to them by the banks), and in the next instant I'd find myself picking them apart.

I thought to myself:

Shad seems great. He's had reported pregnancies and has high-motility sperm. Sure, he's only five feet eight, but I'm tall enough that maybe my genetics could offset that. He's half-Irish and half-Moroccan and has curly, thick black hair and his lips are, sure, "medium." That's still pretty good . . . Not like Davy, with those narrow, thin lips . . . But Shad wears a size eight shoe. Is that thing about shoe size and penis size true? Should I be worrying about my future son's penis size when I choose my donor?! Wait—the bank says he looks like Rami Malek. Hard nope. While an indisputably handsome man, those dead bug eyes kill me . . . (I shuddered after visualizing Rami Malek as a demonic toddler, wide-eyed and obstinate . . .)

Achilles. This is the one. Yeah, his build is listed as "sturdy" (a generous descriptor for heavier donors), *but he's got green eyes. How cool would it be to have a kid with green eyes, like me? Full lips—bonus. Great motility. But . . . ugh. His celebrity look-alike is Vin Diesel and he does multilevel marketing for a living. Hard pass. Thanks for playing, Achilles!*

What about Cort? Sure, he's on the heavy side . . . but he's tall, has full lips, high sperm motility, and reported pregnancies. Wait—he's studying for his MBA and also planning on law school! Damn. My kid could use those brains. The only thing is . . . he's Dominican, Hispanic, and Black. I have zero preference, personally, about my child's ethnicity. But am I equipped to raise a non-white kid in America? Is that fair to the child, when I, a white woman, don't have a partner or co-parent to help them feel connected to their culture and ethnic background? Could that make them feel more "other" when already they come from a single-parent household with no biological father in the picture? Could it endanger their lives if I'm not capable of preparing them for the reality of having a Black or brown body in this country? Damn it. Cort was supposed to be the one . . .

I closed my laptop and glared at Ruby. I had money in the bank, ready to spend on sperm. But something felt off to me about this transaction.

It was maddening. The decision was too important to make based on the limited information available.

On the sperm bank websites, when you're searching for free, you typically get a short bio about the donor's education, hobbies, and basic medical history. Some companies offer short recordings of the donors' voices without the extra cost, usually with the men explaining why they want to donate or describing a relationship that has been meaningful in their lives. For me, it just felt so sterile. There was no way to get a real read on these guys. Plus, they were getting paid—was it just about the money? Could they really be prepared to face my kid in eighteen years, if he or she showed up seeking a relationship? And damn, eighteen years seemed like a long time for that kid to wait for answers.

Shopping for a sperm donor at a bank felt a lot like shopping on Amazon minus the real-world reviews. You often can select several donors and then compare them directly on the bank websites with their key stats listed side by side, including height, weight, and eye color. It was exactly like the product comparisons Amazon offers to allow customers to weigh which humidifier or vacuum they want to purchase. But this was so much more important than the average consumer decision.

It was making me scrutinize the men based on physical attributes as if I were shopping for a designer baby. And that made me feel extremely shallow. And creepy. I care a lot less about hair and eye color—and yes, even lip size—than I do about the kind of person these donors are. And damn my journalistic instincts, but I was having a hard time trusting someone else to do the screening for me. I wanted to *know* this person. I wanted a baby, yes. But it was important to me that the baby grow up to be a kind and happy person. None of this information was going to help me make that happen. I wasn't totally sure what I wanted, but this wasn't it.

Restless, I did what I always did (now that I'd quit smoking) when I needed to think: I took to the streets of Washington, D.C.

I walked mile after mile in my New Balance cross-trainers against the brick sidewalks of Capitol Hill. It had been nearly two hours of striding through the city when the sun finally splashed its pornographic palate across the sky and slid below the horizon, giving me a slight reprieve from the oppressive summer heat. My route had taken me almost full circle back to my apartment when something occurred to me. I stopped short, pulled out my phone, and googled: "sperm donor that you know."

I scanned for a few minutes—enough time to realize that finding a sperm donor who I could actually meet was a thing that could happen. I put my phone away and rushed home.

THROUGHOUT MY TWENTIES AND THIRTIES, especially, I celebrated with my friends as they got married and had children. I attended baby showers with glee, picking out gifts from registries and welcoming new babies with total certainty that my day would come. However, as my early thirties gave way to my mid- and then late-thirties, my ability to feel joy for these momentous occasions had become tempered with anxiety. I resented myself for starting to wonder: *When is it my turn?*

I gravitated toward babies from a young age, and with three younger brothers, I had helped my mom wrangle kiddos for much of my childhood. My connection with my own mother was the singular, most important, formative, and loving relationship I'd ever had, and I wanted to give a child that same sense of unconditional love. I didn't just *want* to be a mom. I was certain it was the reason I was put on earth.

When I found myself single at thirty-eight, something clicked, and I mustered the strength to move forward with becoming a mother without waiting for the "right" guy to come along. Doing it without a partner (whom I would presumably be intimately familiar with) created this unnatural pressure to know *everything* I possibly could about where my baby's DNA was coming from. This was partially for my own peace of mind, but more importantly I wanted to put my future child first.

Despite the unknowns and my brain's relentless onslaught of questions about the process, I experienced a tidal wave of relief after having made the decision about motherhood. I had spent years trying to quash this mommy craving or pretending that the urgency I felt as I aged wasn't a constant buzzkill that I discreetly brought to every first date and long-term relationship, quietly tucked in my back pocket until that moment when I finally dropped the "I seriously need to have a baby" bomb.

I had been successful in my career. It was my personal life that floundered. But everything changed that day in the garden.

I've always been pretty hard-core about my work as a news reporter. I've moved cross-country half a dozen times in pursuit of that journalism dream. Along the way, I've covered all kinds of hot-button issues, including New York State politics, health care, immigration, and the opioid crisis. And I've loved it. As a journalist, you never stop learning new things.

For nearly two decades, the thrill of chasing a story was enough for me. Until it wasn't. I could no longer ignore how unequivocally I needed to become a mom. It was only a matter of time—I had long thought—until I met someone and started a family of my own. But it never materialized. I just never met the right guy.

The first person I told about my decision was my brother Drew. He surprised me with his supportiveness. Not because he's not a supportive guy, but because I was half expecting anyone I talked to about my idea to tell me I was too flaky, too poor, too single to do this whole thing. It felt really good when Drew said that he didn't believe I was totally insane.

"I think you would always try to do your best for your child, which, that's all you can ask of parents, because most parents have no idea what they're doing. But you seem like the type who would do a lot of research to make sure you were being a good parent.

"If you want to have a kid and it's going to make you happy—obviously, you'd be a good mom—then you should do it," Drew told me. "No matter what Mom or Dad says."

"Thank you. I really needed to hear that," I said. I meant it.

Drew was right about our parents. I probably would have pursued single motherhood years ago, but my Catholic mother and father would never approve. I may have been a grown-up approaching my forties, but my parents had always had an out-size influence on my life and life decisions. I actively hid this entire process from them, which was particularly difficult with my mom because we are incredibly close and speak almost daily.

I tested the water, though, one day when I was talking to my mother. I brought up the hypothetical idea of having a baby via a sperm bank. She was quite firm in her opposition. In her words, it was "selfish," because I would be denying the child a father and it would "kill" my own father if I went through with such a plan. That put an end to *that* discussion. But not to my plans.

Fortunately, all my brothers were supportive. Jack, who is ten years younger than me, also brought up my difficulty letting go of my parents' expectations.

"What they think and what they believe really matters to you," he said. "It matters to me, too. But it matters to you so much more in that it affects your whole day . . . Sometimes you get caught up in that. Maybe I'm right. Am I right?"

"You're one hundred percent right . . . And I know they would disapprove. And that's why I haven't done it."

Jack also said he "never had any doubt" I would be a good mom.

"Honestly, I think it'd be great for you as well," he said. "I think you have a lot of love to give, and it would be good for you to have somewhere to put that love."

Again, my brother had touched on something very real. I was happy being single, sure. But there was a void in my life. I needed to be very careful, and honest with myself that I was doing this for selfish reasons. This kid wasn't being asked to be born without a father. I needed to approach my whole plan as thoughtfully and carefully as possible.

FINALLY, BACK FROM MY WALK, I marched across the back patio, flung the sliding door of my apartment open, and lunged for my laptop, landing on the couch across from the fireplace, while only slightly disrupting Ruby. I repeated the Google search that I had started on my walk around the neighborhood.

So many interesting things appeared before my eyes . . . something called the Known Donor Registry, which allows people to search for sperm donors. Facebook groups where sperm donors listed their services—for free? And an app called Just a Baby, where I could swipe left or right on potential donors?!

As I scanned through the various links, a warm sense of certainty came over me. Then I had to suppress a gleeful giggle, because . . . I was definitely going to find a sperm donor on the internet. And that was crazy, but I was going to do it anyway.

This revelation meant that I could stop ignoring the nagging fears and uncertainties that were preventing me from pulling the trigger on a bank donor. When my kid asked me who their biological father was, or why he helped me make a baby, I wanted to have good answers.

This was a path that would allow me to get to know the donor and potentially allow the child to meet him before age eighteen. I could make sure that the biological father of my child was someone I would feel confident introducing to my future kiddo. Even better, I discovered some donors had private Facebook groups for the parents of the donor children to connect so half-siblings could meet each other and have a sense of family.

This was extremely enticing to me as someone who was going to be raising a child without a father. The more family, the more love, the better.

I SOON REALIZED THE WORLD of unregulated sperm donation is as fascinating as it is seedy. In the months that followed, as I interviewed men who had been donating for decades, I learned that the whole movement first emerged on Craigslist and on Yahoo message boards in the early 2000s before migrating to the newer websites and apps of today. Back then, donors would list their availability to donate sperm, and occasionally they would have a taker. Even more occasionally, a woman or lesbian couple would find these online discussions and post that they were seeking a donor. Often these arrangements were anonymous meetups with no way for either party to stay in touch. Sometimes the exchanges involved sex; other times it was just a hand-off of a sterile cup full of sperm in a brown paper bag.

Now, two decades later, unregulated, gray-market sperm donation was exploding online, just as I started dipping my toe in. My reporter senses were set ablaze. This was going to be a huge story. And I was living it. I started taking screenshots of interesting posts on the pages and noting different donors and recipients who seemed to be particularly active in the Facebook groups. I spoke to the people who dominated the world and asked questions as I tried to grasp the nuances of this bizarre social interaction.

Eventually one of the high-volume donors and administrators for several of the groups reached out to me. He saw I was a journalist and said he wanted me to write a story about him.

Sweetheart, I thought, *I'm gonna write a whole damn book.*

But this story is bigger than that donor, me, or any one player. It's about the confluence of demand and supply—especially at a moment when millions of Americans were sitting at home, quarantined during a pandemic with nothing to think about but their mortality. All of these factors spurred an online baby boom.

In 2021, nearly 3.7 million births were recorded in the US—a 1 percent increase compared to 2020, according to CDC data. That may seem small, but keep in mind that the prior five years before this uptick, birthrates were steadily declining by roughly 1 percent a year.

Despite the turnaround, the number of births in 2021 failed to catch up with the 2019 total due to a drop in births between 2019 and 2020.

One of the most popular sperm donation Facebook pages saw its membership grow by thousands per month at times, tripling between June 2020 and June 2022, and eventually reaching about 24,000 members. By August 2023, membership had grown 175 percent. As more recipients flocked to the page, the donor population has grown, too.

One factor that resulted in this boom in the unregulated market is that many fertility clinics closed their doors as "nonessential" medical procedures were put on the back burner during the pandemic, and as sperm banks had to pause accepting new donations—leading to a shortage. Even after clinics reopened, people who couldn't afford to spend thousands of dollars on sperm from a bank, or costly fertility procedures, increasingly went online to find free or cheap sperm. Another upside to a freelance sperm donor is that you're getting fresh sperm (which lives up to five days in a woman's body), and sometimes receiving multiple donations per cycle. By comparison, frozen sperm is almost exclusively administered once per cycle, and it only lives in a woman's body for up to twenty-four hours—making timing around ovulation incredibly critical.

Many of these women, like me, seemed to be in their late thirties and realizing that they were in a now-or-never moment. There's data to back up this existential crisis: In 2021, new births among women ages twenty to twenty-four declined by 3 percent, but they rose as much as 5 percent for women ages twenty-five to forty-four.

Many people gain access to unregulated sperm donation through the Known Donor Registry, a website where donors and recipients can draft profiles and seek each other out. The KDR describes itself as a free community resource and platform for connecting donors and recipients. As such, it has a lengthy "terms of use," in which it makes clear that members are responsible for vetting the accuracy of donor profiles, and for any interaction that may take place. I don't think it's clear how legally binding the terms of use are, but I've heard that people have been kicked off and blocked from KDR for not complying with the rules. The site's code of conduct requires users to be respectful and abstain from using illegal drugs and transmitting STIs. It also recommends legal contracts and bars any requests for payment in exchange for gametes. Members may not "state or imply" that sex is a more effective way to get pregnant than artificial insemination methods.

I found it unwieldy to use the website on a cell phone but appreciated that the site allows users to filter their searches by method of insemination (think: artificial versus sex). In the end, I moved on pretty quickly from KDR because after I created a profile on my laptop, it seemed impossible for me to check or send messages from my phone, which was my primary tool in the search for a donor. I gave up.

I soon started lurking on the Facebook sites and cruising the Just a Baby app, which is like Tinder for getting knocked up. Sperm donors and recipients can post profiles with photos and a brief description, and then they swipe right or left on each other until they find a good match. In my experience, Just a Baby is an extremely unregulated setup. Men who send dick pics or have pregnancy fetishes aren't screened out, so it can require a lot of work for women to filter through those with ulterior motives (though some boldly declare their "preg-fet," donating only to women who will still have sex with them after the second line on the pregnancy test appears). I've found it can also be tough to find a local donor on the Just a Baby app because many of the guys are in far-flung states. Plus, the majority don't include photos or thorough descriptions.

In my experience, Facebook groups are the real lifeblood of this world. Unlike Just a Baby, the Facebook groups allow recipients and donors to exchange information on a semi-public forum, so there's a little bit more accountability. The posts range from insemination advice to pregnancy announcements. Recipients looking for sperm will frequently post a picture along with their location and a few details about what they want in a donor.

Similarly, donors will post photos of themselves and/or their successes. Think: cute baby pictures and positive pregnancy tests. All of this is a bid to attract new recipients.

The groups are also a place where everyone is encouraged to video chat first before meeting in a preferably public place for the first time. The moderators are mostly donors, but there are a few recipients, too.

Moderators do their best to screen out the creeps and trolls. But like any other internet community, I quickly learned that it's tough to keep up with sometimes.

All of this was wildly new territory for me. But there was a palpable sense of empowerment among successful recipients: They had gamed the system, found a shortcut around the reproductive industry, and still wound up with a baby—and a complete family. It intrigued me, particularly in the larger social context of humanity and how we define families. Increasingly, women are becoming parents without a father present, and LGBTQ+ couples are finding ways to build families on their own terms. These online spaces make it possible for many people in marginalized groups to have biological children since the conventional health-care system largely favors coupled heterosexual people with plenty of financial resources.

This is a moment when people are talking more openly about what it means to build different kinds of families and reproductive rights are at the forefront of politics and culture. Along my personal journey, I've explored the psychological, legal, and ethical ramifications of finding free or cheap procreation assistance online and going through with the process of starting a family with the help of a stranger. Could this be a critical moment of empowerment for new kinds of families? Or a risky prospect with myriad complications to consider?

What does it mean if the answer is both?

Either way, more Americans are turning to this world to build their own unconventional families, whether driven by cost, fear of assisted-fertility institutions, or a desire to know the biological other half of their child. Nearly 171,000 American women used sperm from a bank to get pregnant in 1995. By 2016 that number had risen to more than 440,000. As more US women wait longer to marry and have a child, the demand for donor sperm has grown. Rosanna Hertz, author of *Single by Chance, Mothers by Choice: How Women Are Choosing Parenthood Without Marriage and Creating the New American Family,* estimated that approximately 2.7 million American women are single mothers by choice.

Never before have these unconventional paths for building families been more prevalent or compelling. I knew I had to delve deep into this world to learn everything I could about the most unusual road map out there for becoming a parent.

Chapter Two
The Conquistador

*C*ATFISH! *CATFISSHHHHHH,* I THOUGHT to myself.

I had been on the Just a Baby app for less than forty-eight hours before I stumbled across a man with a Clark Kent jaw, paper-cut-sharp cheekbones, and wavy brown hair. He was altogether too beautiful to be real. He also had the sexy cache—and hero status—of being a New York City firefighter. More importantly, he was smart (a degree in business) and had interesting, artistic hobbies, including sculpture. Most importantly, his motivation seemed altruistic. He was only helping people via artificial insemination—and he knew he wanted to keep the number of kids he produced in the single digits. Both of these things were important to me.

I didn't set out looking for a magnificent physical specimen, but it was undeniable. The Firefighter, as I dubbed him, was a friggin' smoke show. Oh Lordy. I could have just as easily called him The Face.

I mustered the courage to swipe right, and we matched. He responded quickly and later that day we video chatted. He was getting off work and still in uniform when he answered my call.

In those first moments, he took off his red firefighter helmet, flipped his hair, and grinned a toothpaste-commercial smile. I was dazzled.

Damn. Those are some good genes, I nearly said out loud.

"Oh! You're real!" I actually did say this out loud, instantly blushing.

We spoke briefly and he agreed to answer my vetting questions via text message and follow-up calls as they occurred to me.

Something happens during the donor-vetting process. It's a way to fast-forward a sense of emotional closeness and intimacy that typically only comes with time, because you're allowed to fire off wildly personal questions with the end goal of partnering to create a human being. Some recipients start to fall for the donor.

My friends were certainly convinced I had the hots for The Firefighter. But it wasn't true. He was five-feet-seven—a full four inches shorter than me. As a romantic prospect, this would be an obstacle. As a potential sperm donor, it didn't bother me in the least. As a relative giant at five-feet-eleven, I figured there was a chance that my genes would ensure any future child was not a shorty. And how much does height really matter, anyway?

I could tell when I spoke about him with my friends that I sounded a bit smitten. I knew my eyes were unfocused and my smile was dreamy as I stared off into the distance or scrolled through his Instagram and the photos he sent me. For the first time I was really able to imagine, with some specificity, what my baby could look like by gazing at his own baby pictures.

The dream was starting to feel more tangible. The Firefighter shared photos from throughout his childhood and of his entire family tree. It gave me a sense of connection that I wanted my child to be able to feel also. He was willing to meet the child and have a relationship, of sorts. But he wanted no legal or financial rights or obligations.

It was a perfect arrangement.

The Firefighter said that he matched with me, at least in part, because of the thought and care I had put into my profile. He said he could tell I was financially stable, had a good head on my shoulders and sincere motivations to be a mom.

I had set about writing my wannabe-mommy ad knowing that I wanted to share a little about myself and what I was looking for so donors would know what kind of person I am and what kind of mother I would be. It didn't take me long to figure out that donors have many options, so I tried to sell myself a bit to attract the most promising candidates. I've heard from a lot of donors that paying attention to things like spelling and grammar is important. Donors should follow the same rules. Some just post a few pictures and their location, like "TAMPA," in all caps. That's not super helpful.

I posted on Just a Baby and later, on sperm donor groups on Facebook:

> Seeking a donor in or near the Washington, D.C., metro area. Artificial insemination only. Will consider working with folks willing to travel. Here's the rub: I'm looking for someone who's willing to be in the kid's

life from birth, not every day or even every week or month. Not a co-parent, but someone who can answer questions for the kid and provide a healthy explanation about why you chose to help their mom bring them into the world.

I'd love to make a new lifelong friend who shares my values and wants to stay in touch, get updates on the kiddo, and attend the occasional birthday party. I'm hoping to find someone reliable and kind.

A little about me: I'm an aspiring single mother by choice. I grew up the oldest of four, and the only girl. I loved caring for my little brothers and always wanted to be a mom. I've just found success in my career as a journalist that has never been matched in my personal life. It is my dream to become a parent, please help me make that happen.

This advertisement, of sorts, won me a ton of matches on Just a Baby, and I was stunned, later, when I received about sixty responses based on that Facebook post. Of those sixty, maybe a dozen men were in my region and four were solid candidates who felt like they had good potential.

Despite crafting an enticing net with my words, plans with The Firefighter ultimately fell apart. It came down to multiple factors. I was hesitant to travel during the pandemic and wanted to find someone who lived closer—for convenience and the possibility that they could be more involved in the child's life.

At the same time, The Firefighter had made a commitment to donate to another couple that had a similar cycle to my own. He couldn't donate to both of us at the same time without, ahem, depleting his reserves.

So we parted ways, and I went back to Just a Baby to start swiping again.

My biggest question through the entire donor search was always: Why do gray-market sperm donors do this? What is their motivation?

Many said they just want to give.

"I do notice a lot of military veterans are donors. So, there's got to be some correlation there, their willingness to help or serve," said Robert, a donor based in the greater New York City-area who asked that I use a pseudonym. He's retired military and still works as a public servant, though he asked me not to specify what his job is now. His first sperm donation helped a friend who was injured in Iraq to get his wife pregnant.

"I've always liked to help people," he said. "I thought he was joking around at first, but I helped them, and they were so happy."

Robert realized there were probably more people out there who he could assist in the same way.

"The banks are very expensive and not very effective," Robert said. "With the Facebook groups they have more of a chance to interact with the donor, their medical background, their likes and dislikes, and all that kind of stuff . . . In this day and age, there's a lot more same sex couples out there and the one thing missing is they want to have a kid together, so I'm willing to help."

He added, "I do have a fee."

The Conquistador

He charges up to $300 for shipping and less for in-person donations. NI donations ("natural" insemination, which is sex) come for free, though he says he stopped offering NI in February 2021. Robert is one of the most in-demand donors on the Facebook pages, largely due to his blond hair and blue eyes—a popular combination among recipients. He often has to turn people away, and says the fee helps him sort out who is serious and willing to follow through; plus he provides all supplies, including a syringe and a menstrual cup to hold the donation against the cervix. Robert is clearly successful: He frequently posts pictures of positive pregnancy tests and of his donor children.

While shipping always comes with some kind of cost (you or the donor can buy kits that include a vial, foam protective packaging, ice packs, and a test yolk buffer, which is a sperm extender that feeds the sperm a nutrient-rich egg yolk from chicken eggs to keep it alive during the overnight shipping process), the vast majority of in-person donations are offered for free. Many donors may prefer NI—one moderator for several of the biggest Facebook groups estimated that 80 percent of all donors on the pages are NI-only donors—but it is possible to find AI-only donors as well.

DeShaun is a donor who chooses not to have sex with recipients because he is in a relationship with a man. He claims to have produced more than 100 children, mostly helping lesbian couples become parents via syringe insemination—though his first recipient had success using an actual turkey baster.

"It makes me happy because I'm helping someone else," DeShaun said. "And I'm helping myself too; if I'm going to ejaculate anyway, it's just going to go down the toilet, so why not help someone?"

DeShaun may appear nonchalant about the fact that he's sired scores of children, but in reality nearly all online donors have their own personal limits and screening processes. Most are concerned about avoiding paying child support or any legal obligation to the child, how likely they are to be successful with a given recipient, and, often, how attractive they find the prospective mother. Some are willing to inseminate everyone and anyone as long as they're hot and willing to have sex (more on this later).

Some specifically ask about what you're willing to do to provide a loving home, which I appreciate.

For example, Tyree is a donor who says he puts a lot of thought into choosing his recipients. He's a thirty-two-year-old father of four from Arizona who says he has been donating sperm through Facebook for five years, producing forty-one children. He said he is popular because many recipients have a hard time finding African American donors at sperm banks. He also seems to attract recipients for being a kind and caring person, posting on his own page about his trips to visit homeless encampments and efforts to bring food, water, and resources to people in need.

"I normally have a list of questions I ask people: Are they able to take care of a new child, are they in a relationship? If they are, are they married? And if they are married, how long have they been married? If they're not married, when are they planning on being/getting married?" he explained.

Donors generally want to know how financially independent recipients are. Some prefer to avoid donating to single mothers by choice, because it's a higher risk than in a two-parent household, in which the non-gamete parent can adopt the child—protecting the donor in the process.

He also asks about their living situation: Do they have a roommate, live with friends, or have their own place? He is excruciatingly aware that some of his recipients could fall on hard times and, while he doesn't think that should preclude them from having a child, he wants to know they will fight to get back on their feet when things get tough.

"One thing I never want to happen is for a recipient to be a burden to the system," Tyree said.

Tyree is taking an unusual step: preparing to adopt one of his donor-conceived children, a two-year-old-girl, along with her half-brother, who is also donor-conceived but has a different biological father. Tyree donated to a married lesbian couple nearly three years ago, but the women have since divorced.

The mother who received sole custody later ended up in jail on robbery and child endangerment charges. Convinced she would never be able to regain custody, she reached out to Tyree and begged him to not only adopt the child who is biologically his, but her five-year-old brother as well.

Tyree didn't hesitate. He immediately contacted child protective services and started the process of asserting his biological parental rights and pursuing adoption of the siblings.

It seems fair and wise for donors to ask careful questions and limit their donations based on a recipient's ability to provide for a child. The handful who I've spoken with who pay child support (including some who have their wages garnished) are the minority, but it's a scary prospect for donors—especially those producing dozens of kids.

Vetting looks different for recipients. Women, first and foremost, should require STI tests from donors. Regular donor STI testing is even more critical for recipients planning to have sex to get pregnant—most NI donors are tested at least every three months, if not more frequently. Donor recipients also often require that a donor undergo genetic carrier testing, which can determine what genetic diseases the recipient and donor could pass on to the child. If both recipient and donor are carriers for the same genetic mutations, it creates a significant risk that the child could be born with that disease. Frequent concerns are cystic fibrosis and sickle cell disease, but there are as many as one hundred to six hundred conditions that genetic tests can pick up on, depending which company and package you choose.

My advice to anyone about genetic testing is just do it, even if you have no reason to suspect an issue. I was shocked to learn through my own testing that I'm a carrier for spinal muscular atrophy, which can be a devastating disease.

No one in my family history on either side has ever had this. Yet I had a very high chance of passing it on to my child if I chose a donor who was also a carrier. The genetic carrier testing gave me peace of mind. It usually costs between $250 to $350, out of pocket. I paid a $100 copay with my health insurance.

Often, recipients also request the donor's sperm analysis, to check the count, motility (meaning how fast and active the sperm are), and the morphology (how uniform and symmetrical the swimmers look) of the sperm. Eventually, I figured out that many recipients skip the sperm test when they're working with a donor who's had a high number of successes.

It's important to note the extensive screening that happens at a sperm bank, which not all recipients in the unregulated sperm market insist on for their donors.

Beyond the potential for sexually transmitted infections, could untested freelance sperm donors—and particularly prolific super-donors—be spreading less than ideal physical and mental health problems?

That's the concern of Dr. Jaime Shamonki, who, at the time of our interview, was the chief medical officer at California Cryobank, one of the largest sperm banks in the country. She is now chief operating officer of US Fertility and Ovation Fertility.

She thinks that even if a woman knows her donor, she should still work out the details through a sperm bank's "directed donor" program so she has access to the other legal protections these companies provide—though that comes at a high cost.

I thought I had checked every box when I had The Conquistador take a genetic carrier test to ensure we weren't both carriers for the same disease. I paid for the cost, and a few weeks later we found out we were genetically compatible—neither of us carried overlapping diseases, so any children we produced wouldn't inherit those traits.

However, sperm banks do more than the straightforward carrier test; it's another level of genetic screening, so detailed that it falls under the purview of a genetic counselor to untangle someone's genetic past and predispositions.

Most people think about genetics in terms of the autosomal dominant disorders, which are genetic traits that, if you inherit them, you will express the trait and there's a fifty percent chance of your child inheriting it as a carrier—unless the biological father is also a carrier, in which case, in addition to the likelihood of being a carrier, the child has a 25 percent chance of expressing the trait. Those aren't ideal odds when the trait is cystic fibrosis or some other life-shortening disease.

If it's up to the average recipient to interview a donor and to try to learn about the importance of his family history, it may not occur to that person to ask if his female family members are carriers of the BRCA gene mutation that is associated with breast cancer.

Unlike the unregulated sperm market, banks also conduct extensive psychological screening of sperm donors to ensure they are prepared for the ramifications of creating a whole new person who could one day have expectations and a feeling of attachment to them. A conversation over a few glasses of whiskey doesn't count as psychological testing, regardless of whether you are someone who generally has good instincts about other people.

Some doctors in the industry—a majority of whom discouraged me and other women to pursue a baby in the unregulated sperm donor market—strongly recommend that the prospective donor get a full health workup.

"There's a lot of risks," said Dr. Allison Rodgers, a Chicago-based reproductive endocrinologist. "If this person is giving you sperm, who else are they giving sperm to? And are they having intercourse with all those other people? And then of course, the psychological evaluation of, is this somebody you're planning on having a relationship with, even if it's from a distance? What is their psychology like—are they doing this for the right reasons? And then the question is, well, what are the right reasons?"

In addition to the obvious need for health screenings, I quickly realized it's a good idea to have a list of questions to get at the heart of Dr. Rodgers's point: What are the right reasons for a person to be donating sperm? A lot of recipients focus on things like height, eye color, hair, or race and ethnicity. Some want highly educated donors or athletic donors. It all depends. I would enthusiastically interrogate my potential donors because who they were as people was the most important factor to me. My kid and I would be tied to this person for life. It was a big decision. To that end, I put together a detailed list of vetting questions, covering family background, medical history, their personality, and the relationship we would have if they were my donor.

Questions included:

- May I see your STI test results?

- Why do you want to donate?

- Please tell me about your family history—physical and mental health on both sides of your family?

- Would you be willing to take a genetic test? Sperm quality/count test?

- May I have more pictures of you, including when you were a baby?

- What kind of relationship would you like with your donor child? How much contact is desirable to you?

- Would you be available to produce future siblings, should I want more children?

- What if you later find out you can't have any more children and still haven't had any of your own? Would that change how you feel about my child?

- What if I die? Would you want custody or first right of refusal?

- Do you stay in touch with other recipients and their children? Are you able to help my child connect with siblings?

- What's your relationship like with your own family?

- Will you sign a contract?

- How many children have you produced from donating? How many do you want to produce by the time you stop?

- What are the genders of your children?

- What are your political leanings?

- How do you feel about your donor children? What would you say if one asked you if you loved them?

- How tall are you?

- Eye color?

- Ethnicity?

- Are you good at math?

- Have you had braces?

- Do you believe in God? Belong to a religion?

- If it comes down to it, would you be willing to still be my donor for in vitro fertilization?

. . .

AROUND THIS TIME, I STARTED tracking my cycle, another important part of the process for recipients. This involves counting from the first day of your period as day one, and then once your period is over, begin peeing regularly on ovulation sticks until they show two lines—indicating that ovulation is imminent. Once I was on track with a clear understanding of what days I would be most fertile, I knew how to time insemination appropriately. Donors often ask to see these ovulation predictor kit (OPK) sticks to get a sense of the recipient's cycle and to avoid wasting a donation on poor timing.

I also had to familiarize myself with the terminology of this community. "AI" means artificial insemination, while "NI" is natural insemination—again, another way of saying sex. Finally, there's "PI," or partial insemination. This is when a donor stimulates himself and then physically penetrates the recipient seconds before climax. I also recently learned of something called "AI-plus," in which the recipient manually stimulates the donor, who then ejaculates into a cup so it can be used for artificial insemination. A lot of donors say that natural insemination is better and more effective at getting people pregnant (I've looked; there's literally no proof of this). Maybe some of them actually believe this, but when they're basically trying to get a hand job out of the transaction . . . it just seems like a problematic proposition, especially when I think about my kid meeting this person someday and trying to understand how and why they came into the world.

Most recipients just want artificial insemination—much to the disappointment of many donors. There are a few ways to perform AI. Many people have the donor produce a sample in a sterile cup. The recipient then uses a syringe to suck up the sample and inject it into their vagina. This process is typically followed by a period where the recipient's legs are propped up in the air, hips angled skyward. Although there's no scientific basis for doing so, it's kind of a tradition on the Facebook pages to kick your legs in the air and post a picture of this moment.

Some recipients prefer to use the "soft cup" or "soft disk" method in which the sample is deposited directly into a menstrual cup, the kind that's designed to fit around your cervix. You then very carefully insert the cup through the vagina, pop it into place, and leave it in for up to twelve hours. The sperm know where to go from there.

AT FIRST, DOWNLOADING THE Just a Baby app and creating a profile felt surreal. It was exactly like a dating app, and that kind of user interface was fairly intuitive, since I'd been on my fair share of dating sites. Initially, it made me feel like I could scan for people without putting myself out there in a more public way, like on a Facebook page.

Once I spent hours swiping—mostly left, which I was also rather familiar with doing—it started becoming more comfortable. I didn't necessarily like using the app, but knowing that these donors were presenting themselves in their own words felt a little more authentic, like a mom-and-pop shop rather than a Walmart. I preferred it to the sperm bank websites, believe it or not, because it allowed me to feel more in control and more confident about making a decision. I realize this path may not be a viable choice, or even a consideration, for many people. For me, it felt less yucky. I don't know how else to explain it.

I soon came across a picture of a goofy but attractive guy about my age. He was bald but very tall, with vivid, cornflower-blue eyes. His profile was brief but seemed genuine. He talked about wanting to help people. He lived about an hour away— much more practical than New York.

I would date him, I thought.

We matched as soon as I swiped right.

Within an hour we were video chatting, giggling about the awkwardness. "You'll be my first," he told me.

"I hope you mean first recipient," I said, accidentally snorting as I laughed at my own crappy joke. He laughed with me.

We met the next day at Mr. Henry's, a classic D.C. haunt where Roberta Flack got her start. Sparks started flying from the moment we sat down in one of the wooden booths and ordered the same whiskey (Jameson). He stood up to greet me as I walked in, and I was pretty sure he checked me out in an approving way. I came prepared with my list of about two dozen questions. He patiently let me rattle them off.

Every answer was exactly what I wanted to hear.

He wanted to become a donor because he wanted to help people, and because for years he had been feeling a biological urge to have children, but recognized he was not in a place where he was ready to do that. He thought being a sperm donor could scratch that itch and he could potentially get pictures, or a chance to meet any resulting spawn. His answer felt honest. His other answers were equally appealing.

Yes, he wanted to be in the child's life. Yes, he would sign a contract and get a lawyer. Yes, he would get genetic and STI testing done. He also agreed to a sperm analysis. Our politics and values aligned. He had a great job that involved a lot of math and science—an attractive genetic contribution that would hopefully complement my own inheritable offerings while offsetting my weaknesses. Yes, he would be open to seeing the child as often as I or the child wanted—say every other week or so. My heart melted at this idea.

When I asked how soon he would want to meet the child, he said, "How soon is too soon?"

"As far as I'm concerned, you're welcome at the hospital—just not in the delivery room." We laughed, awkwardly, and he held my eye contact as we contemplated this.

And he was funny. I asked what the child should call him, given the unusual nature of the relationship. I was fine with his first name, or whatever the donor thought was best.

"How about The Conquistador?" he said, poker-faced. I cracked up, utterly charmed.

Somehow, I got up the courage to ask, "What if the kiddo wanted to call you Dad?"

The Conquistador shrugged. "I'm not going to tell the kid that they can't call me Dad, if that's what feels right to them. I'm not going to, like, reject a kid."

Maybe I should have been more guarded, but my insides immediately turned to goo. This guy was going to be present in the kid's life. This was everything I wanted to be able to give my child.

I was happy to have found The Conquistador, because, even though he hadn't had any successes yet, he didn't plan to produce a large number of children through donation. He didn't have a specific limit in mind but knew he didn't want to hit double digits. That was reassuring.

By the time we left that first meeting, plans were in place to find lawyers to draft a legal contract, and for him to get genetic, STI, and sperm quality testing and analysis. But something was nagging at me: I had a serious crush on my wannabe baby daddy.

Following that initial in-person conversation, we started texting each other twenty to thirty times a day. I was racking my brain to come up with more vetting questions just to have an excuse to talk to him. He reacted with equal enthusiasm, consistently checking in throughout the day and thoughtfully engaging in lengthy conversations. Soon, our exchanges became flirtatious in between planning for the first at-home artificial insemination. It was supposed to be straightforward: He would come over, I would provide him with a menstrual cup, he would use my bedroom to produce a sample in the cup, and he would then leave it for me in the room so I could carefully insert it.

Finally, during all of this planning, he said what we both were thinking: There was something "kinda hot" about the whole thing, about us. Some sexual tension was clearly brewing. This clandestine sexual act—an exchange of fluids while separated by a thin wall—was such a bizarre thing to go through with. We immediately admitted our mutual attraction, which further made this plan weirdly erotic. I was extremely caught off-guard to feel so close to someone (all that damn vetting!) and so turned on by them, so quickly. I had been single for a long time and hadn't been in love for eight years. But I was into this guy. And it felt really good to believe that he wanted me, too.

We decided to meet again to discuss whatever the hell was going on between us.

We acknowledged that it was a ridiculously complicated situation, but we both felt compelled to see where it went. Over the course of an hour and two whiskeys each, we hashed out an improbable and optimistic plan: We would pursue this romantic . . . thing. And simultaneously try to procreate. While also navigating the parameters of him not having any legal responsibility to my future child.

Something made me run face-first toward this highly questionable situation. Still, I tried, in my own way, to protect myself.

I said something along the lines of "Please don't fuck with me or waste my time. I've been through a lot, and I don't need my heart smashed. I am perfectly happy just keeping this a pro-fessional donor-recipient relationship. If we do this, there will be a child involved and it's important that we only do it if we're actually trying for something real and meaningful and long-term. And if it doesn't work out, we have to be mature and get along so we can keep you in the kid's life, because what's best for the future baby is all that matters."

He looked at me with an almost comically serious expres-sion. His hands were clasped in front of him on the table, across from me. His massive eyes looked guileless. He reached across the table and took my hand. I had come across the most date-able, promising, romantic prospect I had encountered in years.

"I haven't felt like this for a long time. I want to see where this goes," he said. "And I think we're mature and well-rounded people who could remain friends, or at least friendly, for the sake of the child if things don't work out."

I believed him as we walked hand in hand back to my apartment for our first attempt at "insemination." I wanted to believe he was romantically interested in me, but a little whisper in the back of my head wondered if he was only interested in the sex. I shushed that voice and squeezed The Conquistador's hand a little tighter.

The Conquistador and I stumbled into my bedroom, slightly buzzed from all the whiskey and unbridled flirting. We undressed each other quickly and clumsily, bumping against the walls of my long hallway. He started whispering that it was going to be so hot to get me pregnant. I played along (as one does) as I led him to the bedroom, and he seemed excited. But when the moment came for him to perform, The Conquistador fell flat. Or flaccid. Naked and drenched in sweat, he apologized.

I tried everything I could think of, but The Conquistador said the stress of not yet having a legal contract in place was a serious distraction.

"Does this happen often?" I asked.

"Yeah, sometimes," he said. I was, unkindly, annoyed by his lack of embarrassment. I was totally unsympathetic, at least in the moment. He had one job. He failed.

I smiled and pretended it was fine and said that I understood. But inside, I was hugely disappointed. First and foremost, this guy was supposed to provide me with a baby. No hard-on, no baby.

He held me for a bit and then said he had to leave. He got dressed as I watched, wrapped in my bedsheet and a cloak of regret.

Then, it happened again. During two subsequent attempts he failed to maintain an erection. I was worried. And extremely turned off. I kept picturing his round, shiny head above me, looking down as beads of sweat dripped off his forehead and plopped onto my pale flesh. His eyes, once so enticing and sweet, looked faraway and almost dissociated from the moment, as he held his soft torso up and gazed down at me from above.

He repeatedly bailed early when we were hanging out and even canceled on me once, blowing off plans when I had made him an elaborate salmon dinner. And let me tell you: When a woman from the Pacific Northwest offers to make you salmon, you don't stand her up.

I was confused. Did he still like me? Did he actually have the romantic feelings he assured me were there? It clearly couldn't be all about the sex since we never got there. What was going through his head? What was he getting out of this? It was excruciating.

Still, we were texting dozens of times a day. He was sweet and kind, and theoretically turned on by the idea of getting me pregnant and having sex while I was pregnant. At one point he sent me porn featuring a very young pregnant woman and an (inevitably) much older man fucking her brains out.

Yes. Clearly, blatant red flags were popping up. But right in front of me was a very tall man who scooped me onto his lap and told me that if things went the way he was hoping, we wouldn't even need the legal contract. My interpretation: He was talking about starting a family with me. Every biological instinct I had suddenly eclipsed my common sense.

Finally, on our third or fourth attempt, The Conquistador managed to stay in the game. I clenched very, very tightly and closed my eyes, psychically willing him to muster what he could to stand at attention. And I am to this day still not entirely sure he wasn't faking, but I thought I felt something. He started moaning as I rocked my hips back and forth on top of him and he let out a little gasp before sinking deeper into the bed with a sigh. Was that it? I couldn't be sure.

The Conquistador

It was the closest we had gotten to creating a baby.

I rolled onto my back and asked him if he came. He said he had. Triumphant delight came over me and I asked him to look away as I inserted a cervical menstrual cup.

My joy at the first successful-ish insemination was short-lived: A week later The Conquistador gave me terrible news. Over text. He had been offered a Very Big Job in another state and was moving on. And he didn't want to maintain anything romantic, let alone produce a child.

A few days later, I got my period.

I felt stupid because I had been stupid. At the time, I felt used. I assumed he must have been acting out a fetish, or at the very least misrepresenting himself and knowingly fucking with my head (after I explicitly and politely asked him not to). He literally called himself The Conquistador. I had been conquered. It was, and remains, humiliating. I treated the world's most bizarre situationship like a relationship. I would never, ever, get romantically involved with a donor again.

Chapter Three
Prolific Producers

ROBERT HAS MADE A RITUAL out of icing his testicles. Every night, he gets two ice packs out of the freezer and inserts them into the appropriately placed pouches on his specially designed boxer briefs. They're the Snowballs brand, advertised as a $59-per-pair solution to help boost fertility. Robert is a faithful customer.

"I do about two hours of that a night," he said. Testicles are "naturally supposed to hang a little bit lower if they heat up so that they can stay cooler than the rest of the body. Icing increases your fertility over time. It doesn't happen right away; but it does boost your testosterone a little bit."

It's a common practice among the most prolific donors. Kyle Gordy, another donor and moderator of many online groups, said he often will ice his testicles while traveling to meet a recipient. He loves to confuse fast-food workers by placing an order and then asking them for a free cup of ice—"for my balls!" He cackles wildly whenever recalling the confusion or alarm on their faces.

Kyle and Robert are part of a small faction of men who make serious emotional, lifestyle, and time commitments to help recipients meet their pregnancy goals. But more than that, they are prolific producers. Kyle and Robert have both fathered so many children that they now seem to give contradictory numbers and undercounts to avoid criticism in the Facebook groups. Or maybe they've lost track.

It's unclear where the line is—what makes a super-donor? A dozen babies? Twenty? Fifty? According to my own anecdotal observations, many donors tend to decide to pursue the lifestyle and become self-described super-donors after producing eight to twelve children. Keep in mind, that may mean they've donated to two dozen or more recipients before actually achieving that number of successes (with every intention to spawn dozens more). Often the rate of success will increase as a super-donor becomes more experienced with timing and the science behind how babies get made more generally—and, some would argue, after they take steps to improve sperm count, quality, and motility.

The super-donors are men who ingest maca root to boost their sperm count and regulate their personal sex lives by abstaining when they have upcoming donations. Some compete with each other for the most children. Or they fixate on the hottest recipients often simply for sex. Many are consumed with producing the best swimmers possible so they can get aspiring mothers pregnant. They build their lives around getting women pregnant, racking up dozens of babies, some even reaching triple digits.

After a long fertility struggle, many women just want a "sure thing."

I've come across several gatekeeping "good guys" in the sperm donor universe. The genuinely decent men say they do their best to keep the creeps out while helping women get pregnant. These are the ones who kept me coming back in search of what I needed.

I've also come across opportunists and scumbags who want to fulfill a particular fantasy, or simply just want sex. This fact is unsettling. In so-called traditional, heteronormative families, there is always the tale of how the mommy and daddy cared about each other so much that they wanted to create a family, and so the child was born of this tender love. It's a much different origin story than that of the donor-conceived.

Susan Golombok, a UK-based developmental psychologist, was part of a team that conducted a survey of donors using a website for recipients and sperm donors to connect with each other. Unsurprisingly, the survey found that heterosexual men were almost entirely motivated by the opportunity for easy sex.

That troubled Golombok, because her work has found that many children often look for meaning in where they came from.

"If they were to find out he just put himself on this website because he wanted to find women who he didn't know to have sex with—I mean, that's not a very nice message about how you came into the world," Golombok said.

LATRICE, A STUNNING AFRICAN AMERICAN woman with long black hair and a penchant for bright red lipstick, had her head on a pillow, her legs in the air, and her toes squished against the ceiling of her bright blue Chevy Equinox.

Her wife had just inseminated her using a "lube-launcher"—a syringe-like device designed to shoot lubricant into a vagina. The couple had traveled an hour from their Michigan home to pick up a cup of sperm from Ron, a super-donor who estimates he's produced sixty-five children and has more on the way.

For three days in a row, they had a conception routine with Ron's help. After picking up the sperm in a cup inside a paper bag from Ron's work space, they would drive a short distance before pulling into a quiet hospital parking lot. Then Latrice laid down and scooted her five-feet-one-inch frame as far into the backseat as she could. Her wife crouched on the edge of the opposite seat, her legs dangling out the partially open rear door. It only took a few seconds for the couple to complete their backseat DIY insemination.

"I kept my legs up for fifteen minutes, then we drove off and went about our day," she said.

The couple hadn't anticipated getting the golden ticket: a first-time success. But a few weeks later Latrice had a vivid dream that she was pregnant. "It felt so real," she said. The next morning, she took a test, and it was positive. Now the couple has an eighteen-month-old son.

Latrice and her wife notified Ron before they told most of their family and friends. They texted him a picture of the positive pregnancy test. He was thrilled for them—plus, it was a first-time success for him, something that super-donors often brag about on the Facebook pages.

Ron says his pleasure comes from the joy he brings recipients when he learns they got that BFP (a big fat positive pregnancy test). While Ron strictly donates through AI these days, it wasn't always the case. For years, he was compelled by an addiction to conception sex.

"I'm fond of saying it's ruined vanilla sex for me—like, just having sex with your partner or lover, or whoever, just for fun. Getting women pregnant became a quest. It is more satisfying when you impregnate a woman naturally. It just flat out feels better," he said.

Ron temporarily stopped donating in 2015, in part because he wanted more pleasure than what could be gleaned from constantly impregnating women through sex. He sought out the help of three different therapists and attended about six sessions with each one. Ron never found the therapy helpful or particularly therapeutic.

But in 2015, Ron had a come-to-Jesus moment after vividly recalling a 1988 trip to the farm country of his childhood. During the visit, he had spotted an old, rust-colored bull named Charlie, whose sole job was impregnating the herd of cows.

The enormous beast (Ron estimates he was six feet tall at the shoulder) was confined, alone, in a fifteen-by-twenty-foot pen and didn't even get to mate directly with the cows. Instead, the farmer's wife handled extracting the ejaculate, and the farmer used it to manually inseminate the cows.

"His life was just to get off and eat and be penned up. And I was like, 'Man, he doesn't even get to roam with the cows, he just is this pent-up animal.' Now, I started thinking, 'Man, I'm just like that bull Charlie. I have no pleasure other than just inseminating women for fun.' And so, I just quit cold turkey."

Ron started thinking more seriously about curbing his behavior after landing in court to answer child support demands. Ultimately, he says, it came down to willpower.

"My lawyer probably was the biggest help," Ron said. "She rather bluntly said, 'You need to stop doing this via intercourse. If for no other reason than, legally, this complicates things for you.' At some point, I just wanted to feel different about myself. And I think it was that internal decision that I made for myself to change."

After that, Ron returned to donating through artificial insemination, and he says his motives are "genuinely altruistic." Ron is open to meeting any donor-conceived children and says he believes DCPs have the right to know their genetic background.

Ron got hooked on donating sperm at age nineteen. He was a college sophomore in the fall of 1987 when his creative writing professor, nearly two decades his senior, introduced him to the idea. She seduced him during a one-on-one session. In the middle of their first tryst, she whispered in his ear that he could climax inside of her—that she wanted him to get her pregnant, no strings attached. He described the resulting orgasm as explosive, life-changing, and the overall experience as formative. It was his first real sexual encounter.

The woman promised him that he would have no responsibility for any resulting child; she was simply running out of time and craved motherhood before it was too late. Ron "donated" his sperm to the professor several more times before the semester ended. He never learned if their efforts resulted in a child.

Ron was absolutely enthralled. Insemination sex became his kink of choice from that point forward; everything else felt bland, he said. He spent years yearning for a similar opportunity, eventually finding himself cruising Craigslist and Yahoo message boards in the mid-2000s, and occasionally finding women who would respond to his posts offering free sperm donation.

Now fifty, he admits that he still finds gratification in the process, and that he gets a little ego boost when he's able to make a recipient's dreams come true. His devotion to the cause often results in strong, trusting partnerships with the recipients he works with—even when problems arise.

Ron had always been a gentleman with Latrice, providing advice and guidance on timing, and never pushed or asked for anything, other than a chance to see the occasional picture and for the kid to have the option to meet him, if interested.

Ron had agreed to help Latrice, and her wife, in part because he simply got a good vibe from her.

"I could tell from her posts that she was a good communicator," he said. "I tend to gravitate toward recipients like that because I know they won't waste my time. She seemed serious and not wishy-washy. And she had her act together."

Latrice's loyalty to Ron was tested soon after she gave birth. The couple had been receiving food stamps for themselves and a fifteen-year-old son Latrice has from a prior relationship. When the new baby came along, the state wanted to know who the father was so that he could pay child support in lieu of the state providing benefits. Latrice said she had no idea who the father was and refused to cooperate with their efforts to locate Ron.

As a result, Latrice's benefits were stripped—an outcome she accepts because it's better than the alternative of betraying her donor. The couple are planning to work with Ron again in 2024 to have another child.

"He gave us the best gift," she said. "We had an agreement, and I won't go back on that."

THE MOST VISIBLE SUPER-DONORS TEND to be leaders in the online sperm community. They moderate groups, start conversations, and maintain visibility by regularly posting about their pregnancy successes.

This is both good and bad. Super-donors bring the commitment that is required to manage these pages around-the-clock. However, complaints have arisen among the women in the groups about how these super-donors handle problematic men. The men who run the group ask that any donors behaving inappropriately be reported to them; they then investigate and, if needed, remove the person from the group and notify leaders of other groups. (Many administrators and moderators oversee multiple groups, even a half-dozen or more.)

However, the group leaders don't allow recipients to post the name and photo of problematic donors to warn other women not to work with them. Sometimes it's just a donor who is scamming women out of money, but other times it's allegations of sexual coercion, or discovery of a donor's criminal record. Perhaps this is why, in my three years immersed in this world, I've never once spoken to a woman who had gotten an STI or been sexually assaulted—but it doesn't mean it hasn't happened.

Women have been kicked out of the groups for putting these bad-actor donors on blast. The super-donor moderators do this to keep complaints quiet so they can control the narrative by trying to keep online conversations and posts on-message: The Facebook groups are safe and better than sperm banks. Anything contradicting that message gets quashed. It was something I couldn't get vocal about throughout my reporting process without risking being cut off from the groups. Bottom line: At times when it really counted, the moderators protected their ability to continue donating instead of protecting the women in the group.

Rose Marie knows all about the creeps. She's a single mother by choice and one of the outlier women who has stuck around to moderate several donor groups—and she's seen many screenshots of conversations from potential recipients in which the super-donor is attempting to manipulate the recipient into sex.

When this happens, Rose Marie will contact the donor to firmly remind them that it's against group rules to pressure anyone to pursue methods other than what the recipient is seeking. Periodically, admins will post group public service announcements reminding everyone of these policies, but it seems like a constant battle for them to get men to stop crossing that line. Men have gotten angry at me for turning down their request to provide natural insemination. Usually, the conversation starts out normal enough, even carrying on for several days of going through various vetting questions. Then it can turn creepy. Some donors seem to feel that recipients owe them sex. The repetition of constant, unnuanced sexual overtures got old very quickly. It started to seem like guys were playing a numbers game: ask for sex from enough women, and eventually someone is going to give you what you want.

Early on in my days on the Facebook groups, I noticed some men would call "dibs" when an attractive woman posted a photo of herself seeking a new donor. Eventually, the moderators got a grip on the whole thing because women were getting so disgusted, they were threatening to leave the group.

But the fact that it happened in the first place burned into my mind that many men were here to get off.

A handful of longtime super-donor moderators have repeatedly been accused of getting competitive by punitively banning new, good-looking donors or those who are geographically positioned to compete with them directly among local recipients.

Complaints periodically pop up about the Facebook groups seeming to limit allowing new donors in, but most were too nervous to go on the record about it.

"It's not okay, if, say, you're in Los Angeles, to try to be the only Los Angeles donor just so that you can, like, clean up and get some," one donor said. "The recipients may want different things. And that's okay; a woman might reasonably want different things."

This was likely a reference to Kyle, who is known to have a stronghold over many of the most popular sperm donation groups on Facebook. Kyle denied that he, or other moderators, has kept people out of the group for competitive reasons.

Kyle was technically banned from New Zealand, Australia, and even Canada—where he was questioned for four hours, after admitting on immigration documents in New Zealand that he was a serial sperm donor (he suspects New Zealand shared the records with the other two countries).

Super-donors in control often don't like to let new donors who could compete geographically or genetically into the group. Considering the high populations in California and New York City—where two of the most prolific donor/moderators live—

there seems to be disproportionately fewer donors from those areas than one would expect. In my observations, a moderator who is, say, a white guy, might allow an Asian donor who is also based in the same region to join the group. But this same super-donor would be unlikely to let another local donor in who was also white, with desirable traits like being over six feet tall with blue eyes. Part of the problem is that women join the groups, get pregnant, and leave. Nothing will change until women lay claim to more permanent moderator roles or create their own groups with some minimal screening of donors.

At one point, it came out in the groups that a popular donor was also a convicted sex offender. He had red hair and blue eyes, a popular combination that had produced an estimated twelve children, according to a few people who said they knew him before he was outed in the groups. The woman who posted his mugshot and sex offender registration page in the main Facebook groups was kicked out and had her post taken down. The admins didn't want anything posted that ran contrary to the narrative that freelance sperm donation was a safe, better alternative to sperm banks. They put their ability to donate (and, often, to get laid) before the safety and well-being of the women of the group and the children they would create.

One recipient, who uses the pseudonym Melissa, had an experience traveling to meet a donor who promised her that he would do AI, but when she arrived, he said it had to be NI or nothing. She refused to have sex with him but lost out on the cost of the motel room and gas money for driving six hours, plus a wasted cycle without a pregnancy. She also traveled for a donor who she later learned was donating to multiple women—depleting his reserves instead of abstaining and timing donations accordingly.

Fortunately, there are good guys out there.

Stephanie Wicker's donor has been a positive presence in her toddler son's life since birth. Wicker has carefully nurtured a relationship between her new family of two and her donor and his wife—with everyone focused on what's best for the child.

"Initially, I wasn't sure what that relationship would look like," said the nurse practitioner and single mother by choice, who found her donor online. "But it has evolved into regular updates with my donor and his wife. It has also allowed my son to get to know his half-sister [from another single mom by choice]."

She is prepared for the relationship to continue to evolve once her sperm donor and his wife have children of their own. "But it's been really great so far, just to build this nontraditional family," Stephanie said.

Like me, Stephanie believes that more focus needs to be placed on the experience of donor-conceived people—and their perspective must be used to shape the future of the donor-gamete industry.

Some super-donors insist they can maintain relationships with all of their children—even Ari Nagel, who is forty-eight years old and has produced 142 children to date, in countries across the globe, with 15 more on the way. "Sometimes I went to other countries, and I had to actually marry the woman so that we were able to go to the fertility clinic; it was very, very tedious," Ari said. "Other times, when women needed IVF or other medical intervention, we had to travel to another country, because the country where they were required a marriage. I've done all of that."

He periodically posts pictures on Facebook of his globe-trotting to help more recipients. Ari said his motivation and satisfaction comes from helping others.

"I enjoyed being a father. So, when a lesbian couple asked me for help to grow their family and then at the same time, there was also a single woman that asked me (to donate) because she wanted a child, it just felt like a good idea."

Ari said initially he felt a drive to grow his own family and procreate beyond what he could provide for in his regular life as a college professor. Now that he has so many children, he says his motivations are more altruistic than when he first started.

Ari believes super-donors fulfill a need, even as what he's doing remains taboo.

"I think a lot of people's perception is 'Why don't they just adopt?'—not realizing the challenges associated with that," he said. "And I think people feel like, 'Well, why don't they just go through a clinic?' Not realizing how awkward it is to choose the father of your child without having known them.

"Normal [sperm bank donation], to me, sounds crazier," Ari said. "The most important decision in your life is really being made with you going in blind."

By comparison, Ari's recipients can see pictures of children he's already produced, find out if they have any genetic health issues, and even meet some of the other recipient parents to get a general vibe check.

VERY SOON AFTER STUMBLING ACROSS the Facebook community and posting a profile offering his sperm, Mike was inundated with messages. It was a tidal wave of women who wanted to choose him, and that was utterly unlike anything he had experienced in the dating world. In this new, very specific way, he was desirable. And it felt good.

"Next thing you know, I have women saying, 'Yeah, I want you to get me pregnant,'" Mike said. "We got together, and we did it, and it was that simple, really."

Mike says he didn't have a fetish initially, but he now considers baby-making sex the most enjoyable kind of sex. As a sperm donor he's able to have sex with more women—and more attractive women—and it's more gratifying because it has a purpose. For Mike, sperm donation satisfies a primal need he can't seem to shake.

But Mike now no longer craves sex for sex's sake, or in the context of a relationship. It's only meaningful, interesting, and enjoyable if the purpose is to get a woman pregnant. He, like many of these men, seems to become less capable of interacting with women in general. He appears to cling to the hope that creating a child with these women could somehow lead to some future relationship or connection.

Mike is close with his parents and is just starting a career after graduating from college. He's been donating for about three years and has produced at least nine donor children so far (not all recipients tell donors when they conceive).

"Even for the guys who are in this purely for sex, it is still a fair trade. You know, these women want to get pregnant, and a guy wants to have sex, and it makes sense that you would do both at the same time," Mike said.

Dr. Monte Miller, a New York City–based psychologist and sex therapist, said he isn't deeply familiar with the underground sperm donor marketplace but that an obsessive breeding fetish is often about men exerting dominance over women, particularly when consent isn't central to the sexual trysts.

I KNEW I DIDN'T WANT to work with a super-donor. I felt uncomfortable with the idea of my kid having dozens of siblings and a biological father who could never make time to forge a meaningful relationship of any kind.

Plus, I found these men's compulsion to spread their seed far and wide almost pathological. Many spoke of living double lives, keeping their clandestine trysts and donations a secret from everyone who knows them in their "real" lives. It seemed this was at once thrilling—they were living out their ultimate fantasies—and constraining. Many of them use fake names for fear of being discovered for what they are: serial sperm donors consumed with spreading their DNA.

Super-donors also come with a risk that not all recipients may be considering, said I. Glenn Cohen, a bioethicist at Harvard.

"The concern is the problem of accidental incest, which is a bigger problem in places like Iceland, which are smaller and choose less heterogeneity in terms of who marries who, and who has sex with who, but it's a real problem," Cohen said.

I haven't found any actual instances of this, but that hasn't stopped bioethicists from pondering the possibilities. It did become a concern in Oregon when one man—who had been promised by a bank that his sperm would only be used to produce five children—learned that he had at least nineteen biological offspring in a small geographic area.

Another potential issue is that the more children a super-donor produces, the less time, attention, and emotional capacity they have to eventually meet with each individual kid who comes knocking on their door.

I was curious: How do these donors and super-donors feel about their children? Do they love them? One donor said that he loves all his children—to the extent that he feels drained emotionally by the burden of fracturing his love into dozens of pieces, as he can't turn off the emotional connection he feels. But he was the minority. Many super-donors said they feel more for their children than they do toward a stranger's child on the street—but it's not love.

"I don't think with any of my kids that it's a connection where I'm like, 'This is my kid, I have to do everything for this kid,'" said Kyle, one of the most public and self-promotional donors in the freelance sperm world. He says he's produced sixty-five children so far, though after some backlash on the Facebook groups against high-volume donors, he's been more tight-lipped about his latest numbers.

While Kyle says he likes all the kids he's helped produce, he doesn't spend time with them, provide care for them, or forge an emotional bond. He doesn't see himself as the father of any of these children. In most cases, that's how the recipients want it.

"I have to look at it this way; these kids are still the kids of the parents who take care of them. I'm the donor," he said.

Other donors have said they do love their donor children. One thirty-year-old donor, who goes by Jacob, described sperm donation as an almost painful gift, because he loves his donor kids so acutely that every one of them walking around has taken "a piece of my heart," and the process of loving these little people he will never get to know has eroded his own sense of wholeness.

Jacob is particular about to whom he will donate. He will only help prospective parents who agree to loosely stay in touch and be honest with the child about their conception. He's also tried to raise awareness among his fellow donors about the importance of keeping the door of communication open for all donor-conceived children.

Jacob estimates that roughly 10 percent of the recipients have never come back to him. Many send yearly updates, photos, or videos. Some of them are kind, friendly, and make him smile. He's also friends with some of the mothers on Facebook.

"I can occasionally see when they upload a photo or video of the child. I totally understand that they have their own lives, and I don't want their friends or family to become suspicious. I just try to observe from afar, try to be discreet. I don't want to ruin their life."

SOME DONORS HAVE EXPRESSED CONFUSION about what it means to be a man, particularly in the post-#metoo era—a period in which the word "masculinity" is rarely heard without the word "toxic" directly preceding it. The younger donors, in particular, wrestle with knowing how to interact with women. The struggle is particularly acute among those who don't remember a world before the internet, on-demand porn, or the swath of social media platforms that have only made real-world social fluency rarer.

Sperm donation is an incredibly masculine act for some of these guys, and it comes with the added benefit of being a social transaction where the expectations are clear-cut. And the community that these men have forged has also allowed them to create new outlets that many feel are positive.

"A lot of the old walls of the boys' clubs are breaking down," said Gideon, a pseudonym for a popular super-donor. "What is attractive about this sperm donation world is that once you get to know some other donors, you realize they have the same problems you do. When you're in this kind of quasi-secret society of Facebook super-donors, a place not known to the rest of the world, it allows you—ironically—to chat with another guy about something that might be truly embarrassing, or being in a fragile mental state, or feeling vulnerable."

Gideon was worried that if he spoke to me that I would liken all donors to men's rights activists—a comparison to which he would take offense. He believes certain spaces should be preserved for only women and only men, and that gray-market sperm donation has allowed for the simplicity of shared experiences to bring men together.

"It's a funny type of bizarre male bonding," Gideon said. "I wanted to make kind of a cool-guys club, in a sense. Now that I've had success, I want to promote other guys who I think are good people."

Gideon was the closest I got to inside the mind of a serious sperm donor. He gave me confidence that there were genuinely "good guys" out there. He opened my eyes up to another element of this bizarre subculture: It's also a space where men can come together to form friendships, and generally be masculine without fear of repercussions. While these friendships stay almost entirely online or over the phone, many men have described an appreciation for a sense of belonging that has emerged from the groups.

Gideon says they talk about donation, including the standard discussions around supplements and other methods for increasing sperm count and improving motility. He claims they also talk about hobbies, sports, the stock market, or even the odd Broadway musical.

Gideon, who is in his early forties, says he's coached many of the younger donors, who seem to struggle even more with understanding and navigating their masculinity, on how to appropriately interact with women. The prevalence of pornography among younger donors has given some a warped sense of what healthy sexual relationships look like, or what women actually want and enjoy. These groups provide a space where these young men can ask questions, seek advice, and find themselves getting good-natured chiding from the group when they are out of line—at least that's what Gideon tells me. I'm excruciatingly aware that there's only so much access I will be granted.

Gideon wasn't afraid to discuss the problematic men and guys who couldn't seem to stop inboxing women with gross comments.

"I don't want to disparage," Gideon said, explaining that he has had to tell some newer donors to stop commenting on every woman's post that they were "available for NI."

I found this completely obnoxious and said so.

"I would rather take the chance to mentor someone," Gideon countered. "You know the joke about men and parking spaces?" He waited a beat. "The good ones are taken, and the rest are handicapped. Well, some of these gentlemen are handicapped with their social skills. And that's probably why they looked into donating."

He acknowledged that some donors are "uncoachable," and he's worried those men will give the unregulated sperm world a bad reputation.

"There are women who want families that can't afford a sperm bank, and who would do a good job as a mom. And they may see these uncoachable donors and say, 'Oh, yeah right.'"

He even explained his own logic behind the entirely unsubstantiated theory that many NI-only donors push: Sex is more successful than artificial insemination. In Gideon's words, it comes down to volume.

With sex, "you're more aroused, your blood is pumping . . . You're going to not come as much when it's just like a random, forced ejaculation," Gideon said.

Gideon is popular, largely due to his resume: He's over six feet tall. He's bald but had blond hair before he started shaving his head. He has blue eyes, was a college athlete (wrestling and football), is well-educated, and has a job in the field of science. He also has many pregnancy successes. He's quite the character, writing new lyrics to popular songs using the theme of sperm donation.

Gideon now charges typically $100 to $200 for donations, because he's been ghosted by a number of recipients and finds that doesn't tend to happen when they have financial skin in the game. It also helps support the cost of supplements and feels like financial compensation for the time spent moderating

Facebook pages and coaching recipients who are unfamiliar with tracking their cycles.

Gideon also seems to genuinely enjoy helping people, and tends to hold the hand of his recipients, coaching them through the process and working with them to make their baby dreams happen.

"What makes people happy is having the chance to have a family," he said, adding that people should have the ability to choose between a sperm bank or a freelance donor—and not just based on cost.

Being a donor has affected his lifestyle in several ways, though he doesn't take as many supplements or restrict his diet as much as some of the more zealous super-donors.

"I would eat a lot more hamburgers if I were not donating," Gideon said. "And white bread and stuff. Because if you're lifting then you can tolerate anything because it will kind of get you more gains in the gym, as they say. But if you're donating, you don't want to try that. Because it's going to set off more insulin response, which may hurt or harm your sperm."

Donating has affected his life in other ways. His sex life, specifically. Having to ejaculate on demand, and getting to periodically have sex with new women, makes it harder to connect in the dating world. I sensed a longing in him, a craving for human connection that is more than just donation. Perhaps it's safer for Gideon and men like him to get their needs fulfilled with sperm donation because it allows them to avoid the gamble of rejection and even heartbreak.

"I'm thinking back to where I was, before I was donating and just dating. It maybe messes up your junk, you know? It's harder to get aroused almost now. It's also why I stopped looking at porn for the most part. I'd rather just use my imagination because it kind of desensitizes you. There's something in the way it wires your dopamine system . . . It may take me forever to get ready, because you're doing it like it's a job."

When Gideon does engage in NI, he says he tries to set the recipient at ease.

He tells me that he usually starts with the music, something not too romantic but with a sensual vibe—think Cigarettes After Sex. Then he dims the lights, busts out some candles, and tries to joke with the woman, encouraging her to slow dance with him. All of this may be happening in her home, or a motel room, somewhere they've agreed to meet up. The pseudo-romance of the situation seems to make it more meaningful, or at least comfortable, for him too.

Gideon has been in such high demand that he's periodically felt depleted (in more ways than one) from back-to-back donations, day after day.

"I like the build-up and the eroticism, all that kind of thing . . . I'm not just trying to get off anymore now that I'm in my forties. Masturbating and ejaculating for a donation just feels kind of empty," he said, adding that it can feel "life-force draining. I joke it's like being a sex worker."

Gideon also said he often fulfills the recipients' fantasies as much as they fulfill his—and that a common misconception is that only men crave conception sex.

Sometimes, Gideon says, a woman will desire the sexual encounter even more than she wants the baby.

"This woman may just like the thrill, the idea, the fantasy, of this handsome gentleman impregnating her or making love," he said.

Chapter Four

The Lawyer

I DIDN'T LET MYSELF THINK about it. I used one hand to pull down my pants, while the other carefully nestled the cup of fresh sperm, which felt oddly warm in my palm. I took a deep breath, braced my neck and upper shoulders against the wall, and sank down while walking my legs out in front of me, thrusting my pelvis forward to get them as horizontal as possible.

For a moment I slipped a few inches and almost fell. Adrenaline immediately coursed through my veins; my brain shrieked—*Don't spill the sperm!*—but I recovered. I pinched the menstrual cup closed, slid it inside my vagina, and popped it into place against my cervix.

I had done it. Insemination in a public restroom. This was really happening.

I stood up straight and (enthusiastically) washed my hands. A weird tingly feeling came over me as I imagined the sperm working their way through my body and visualized a plump, healthy egg just waiting for their arrival. *I could get pregnant.*

All of this was made possible, of course, by my new donor: The Lawyer.

I was still in my early days on the Facebook pages—and pretty much fed up with Just a Baby—when a local man reached out to me after seeing some of my comments and activity within the groups.

He was an attorney with a professional approach to donating, with his own contract already drafted and a list of his own questions—many about my ability to provide for the child. He was pleased with the thought I had put into motherhood, and that I was financially stable. The Lawyer also asked about my family and how supportive they were. He asked about my physical and mental health, and if I smoked or used drugs. He wanted to know if I had thought through how circumstances in my life would change once a baby arrived, as well as get a feel for my personality, interests, and values. The Lawyer did most of his donating on the Known Donor Registry, but had recently moved to Facebook, as that's where most of the activity had drifted since the pandemic started.

He seemed like a bit of a nerd, but in the best possible way. He had made all the responsible choices in life, in terms of where he went to school and the career he chose. He was thoughtful and inquisitive about my cycle, how many children I ultimately wanted, and how I envisioned parenthood. He had almost as many questions as I did—which he answered patiently, first by phone, and then via Messenger over the next several days.

No, he didn't want to have dozens of children. Yes, he was willing to stay in touch to share any health information that could have genetic components. We shared the same political views, and he was able to speak extensively on matters of global and domestic importance. Yes, he was willing to donate via AI and wouldn't pressure me for sex. He had a fiancée who knew he was a freelance sperm donor, and she had no problem with it. He also had a very slow rate of adding families, ultimately ending his donating with me, with his total around ten families created. His reason for donating seemed legit. He had learned about how expensive it was to buy sperm, but other factors inspired him as well.

The Lawyer had pale, olive-toned skin, brown wavy hair, medium brown eyes, and a charming, mischievous, Cheshire cat mouth that just barely curled up at the corners when he grinned.

He grew up as an only child; his mother had him when she was thirty-nine. His parents had dreamed of giving him at least one sibling, but they gave up after several miscarriages. He remembers the last miscarriage his mother had, when he was in first grade, and the devastation it caused her.

That experience stuck with him and informed his own approach to donating, and he realized he could make a difference in the lives of those families. This made him feel good—he wanted to help people. He also felt a biological imperative to procreate.

"As a normal person, you only get to conceive in a relationship with so many kids in your lifetime. But this kind of gave me the opportunity to experience this before I would be doing that—and more than I normally would, otherwise.

"It's kind of a high getting a positive pregnancy test," he said. "I love it when I see photos of my donor kids and I get their good news."

He had eight successful pregnancies and births by this point, with one of the children born as a sibling into a family he had already helped. The pictures of the babies he'd produced were absolutely adorable, and he had a Facebook group where the moms had the option of connecting and meeting each other. This last part was particularly appealing to me. I wanted my child to be able to know his or her siblings, and to be able to connect, myself, with other mothers who had chosen the same path.

Our first in-person meeting was a bit odd, courtesy of the pandemic. I had been pacing nervously outside the front doors of his swanky apartment building when he appeared, wearing a medical-grade mask that made it hard to tell if he was really the guy from the pictures. When he spoke, he sounded like Darth Vader with postnasal drip. I wore an Etsy cloth mask with bright flowers and paisley, which was clearly designed for form over function. It was September 2020, and everyone was braced for the next wave of COVID-19 to sweep through the nation that winter, again snuffing out lives and leaving grief wherever it struck. I couldn't blame the guy for being extra cautious.

We rode the elevator, awkwardly exchanging muffled small talk about the weather and the damn coronavirus before exiting on the second floor, which was an open office space for residents of the building who wanted to work or hold meetings there. It was eerily quiet. We were the only ones on the floor, except for a cleaning lady who was diligently disinfecting chairs that looked like no one had ever sat in them. We sat down in a booth across from each other and pulled out the tentative contract. We were preparing to exchange bodily fluids, yet we hadn't really even seen each other's faces.

We had already gone through the various terms, one by one, talking through what we needed and wanted out of the situation. He let me ask him, a more experienced player, about his own perspective on the world of underground sperm donation.

"What do you think about the other donors in the group? From my perspective, and from women I've talked to, there's a lot of creeps," I said.

"Every other donor I've seen, from my impression, has some selfish interest in doing this. Some donors charge for their donations. And that might be part of their self-interest," he said. "A lot of them do okay financially, they don't need to charge two or three hundred dollars, or whatever it is that they ask."

"But so many donate for free, and many will agree to do AI, even if they prefer to have sex. What's that about?" I asked.

"The issue is that they want to have lots of kids out in the world, and part of me gets that," he said. "Even apart from the sex aspect of it . . . If I were to be hit by a car on my way home, hey, at least my genes are going to survive."

Yet The Lawyer still likes to differentiate himself from most other donors, particularly the super-donors who tend to control the Facebook groups and engage in regular outreach to the press for attention in the media.

The Lawyer also has major concerns about sperm banks, and views helping women avoid them as an ethical and karmic win.

"It's less effective. It's more expensive. They don't do any actual research into the backgrounds of donors," he said. "I could go through the long list of reasons. I don't think if a woman needs a donor that it should be a bank or nothing."

I appreciated his honesty on everything. This was the kind of easy, transparent conversation I wanted to have with a donor. The only challenge was that he didn't want to meet the child until he or she reached age eighteen.

Otherwise, he was perfect.

I understood his thinking. He had produced more children than he could reasonably be a father to and didn't want to hurt them by refusing to take on the role of Dad. He didn't want to be in a position of rejecting a child, or letting them down because he wasn't able to fulfill the role of a father by, say, attending school events, or playing a hands-on role. This fear was particularly acute because many of the women he donated to (though he was quite tight-lipped about the other recipients) were also single mothers by choice. That comes with more risk than donating to a couple. He believes children are more capable of handling the unusual dynamics of meeting their donor at eighteen than they are before that age. He was afraid that anything he did—even benign kindnesses or small gifts—could later be perceived as father-like by the kids, also making it easier for recipients to pursue child support.

We compromised: He agreed to accept and respond to letters from the child prior to age eighteen to address questions he or she may have. And he would keep his mind open to meeting the child in their later teens if appropriate boundaries were established.

Once it was settled and the contract was signed, it was time to do the insemination. We were still waiting to get his genetic test results back but decided to roll the dice and get started. Later, we learned that he was not a carrier for spinal muscular atrophy, which had been my main concern.

It was at his apartment building, on that floor with the open-concept office space, that I attempted my first insemination.

The Lawyer went into the men's room while I waited, mask-clad, on a couch nearby. After about twenty minutes he messaged me that he was ready, so I met him by the door, took the sample, and slid into the ladies' room. I locked the door behind me and looked at the soft cup full of sperm. This was weird. This was so utterly weird.

It was showtime.

"I DON'T NEED A MAN. I need a strong support system," said Gloria, the pseudonym for a thirty-seven-year-old aspiring single mother by choice who found her sperm donor on the Known Donor

Registry. She grew up in religious household, and pursuing the solo mom route was—whether she liked it or not—a profound act of rebellion.

She went through a long-term relationship with a guy she met in her early twenties. The relationship eventually turned abusive. It took her two years to recover from the trauma of that experience.

"This isn't something where you wake up one day and just say 'I'm gonna have a baby on my own,'" Gloria told me. "For me, it's been a five-year journey. It's definitely a process that you go through and it's a conscious decision. And it's challenging and it's emotional."

I related to Gloria on every level. At this point I was approaching a dozen cycles of home insemination with The Lawyer. The road is long and filled with potholes, misleading traffic signals, and many terribly distracting roadside attractions. Gloria got it. She was ahead of me on the same path.

"My journey has actually been a lot about falling back in love with myself," she said. "Knowing what I deserved in a husband or a partner. I'm learning how to set boundaries and protect myself and creating a space not just for me, but also my son's family and potentially another child." Gloria had endured two decades of relationship disappointments, and as a result, she was ready to let go of the traditional family narrative that said she must couple with a man to have a family.

As she embarked on the solo parenthood path, she thought carefully about the fact that her child wouldn't have a father. It wasn't something she took lightly.

"You can provide a very healthy environment with a strong male role model and female role models in their life without actually being in the traditional structure. And who knows? I hope that I find a partner at some point in time, but by the time I do I probably won't be fertile."

Like me, Gloria was worried about how the absence of a biological father in the household could affect her child. Then she remembered her own father, who, while a good person, wasn't around much.

"He was at work sixty hours a week. And I think a lot of people can relate to that. And that's why the role of a father is so important, but it's not everything."

She chose her donor carefully, had a "very intentional" checklist. She wanted someone emotionally mature, with enough experience donating sperm to make her feel comfortable with the process. She waded through a few interviews with donors who didn't strike that comfortable balance between experience and obsession.

"With this donor that I ended up with, I just got on a call with him, and I instantly felt calm and peaceful . . . He's done a donor screening with a psychologist. I liked that . . . I liked his genetics, that there weren't any issues there. He does not drink or smoke. He tends to look after his body. And I liked that he has been working with a fertility specialist. He has done a lot to do this. And he also did it to have a personal connection. That's how he got into sperm donating."

Again, like me, it's important to Gloria that her kid can meet his or her donor without having to wait until age eighteen. She put thought into the fact that as kids enter their teenage years, they start to establish a more independent identity. Where we come from becomes important at that phase of life.

"I wanted to leave that option open for this child to be able to reach out and get some answers and ask questions at a younger age," she said. "Who knows what's going to happen? Maybe I meet my partner and get married, and my child never wants to meet the donor . . . But I don't have a right to make that decision for them."

In the end, Gloria views the prospect of solo motherhood, and finding a donor she knows on her own, as a story more about personal empowerment than one of compromise or grief over the lack of a father for her child.

"I, as a woman living in America, have this choice. I have a freedom to make this choice. And I don't have to be forever tied to someone like a partner that I don't love or respect or honor."

Again, like me, it's important to Gloria that her kid can meet his or her donor without having to wait until age eighteen. She put thought into the fact that as kids enter their teenage years, they start to establish a more independent identity. Where we come from becomes important at that phase of life.

"I wanted to leave that option open for this child to be able to reach out and get some answers and ask questions at a younger age," she said. "Who knows what's going to happen? Maybe I meet my partner and get married and my child never wants to meet the donor . . . But I don't have a right to make that decision for them."

In the end, Gloria views the prospect of solo motherhood, and finding a donor she knows on her own, as a story more about personal empowerment than one of compromise or grief over the lack of a father for her child.

"I, as a woman living in America, have this choice. I have a freedom to make this choice. And I don't have to be forever tied to someone like a partner that I don't love or respect or honor."

GLORIA AND I HAD MORE in common than our solo motherhood dreams. Raised Mormon and from Utah, she came from an extremely religious family and was keeping her plans to get pregnant a secret from her parents. She hasn't figured out how or what she will tell them when she gets pregnant and starts to show. The hope is that once a child comes along, the acceptance will follow.

This entire time I've also kept my journey a secret from my Catholic mother, who is usually my confidante and my cheerleader. I definitely want her in my child's life, and was also hoping the reality of her first grandchild might be more powerful than her disappointment in my path. I couldn't imagine her not being heavily involved with my child. Babies—just random babies in strollers on the street—will openly giggle in delight when my mother smiles at them. They stop crying when she picks them up. She is radiant with love. I would need her support.

As my heart broke every day after every unsuccessful cycle, I couldn't tell my best friend. I couldn't cry to my mom. It was the most alone I have ever been.

Further complicating the situation is that my mother is married to my father, with whom I had a falling-out right as I decided to pursue motherhood. We have not spoken in years now and have long had a difficult relationship. The first time he stopped speaking to me was when I decided to live "in sin" with my boyfriend at age eighteen. I couldn't imagine the level of disapproval this new motherhood decision would reach on my father's disappoint-o-meter. And if I did tell my mom, it would put her in a difficult situation.

But so much of this situation was part of a bigger phase of my life, in which I was stepping out of the shadow of what my parents thought. I'm going to die one day. I need to live my life for me, chase the dreams that will make me happy.

The fact is that I've always sensed that my dad is ashamed of me and disappointed in how I turned out because I'm not Catholic and I didn't wait until marriage to have sex (or ever get married), and because I'm a journalist for the mainstream media—which he views as an enemy of the American people. We have very different beliefs and values.

I refuse to let that disappointment or shame have any power over me any longer. Having a child is the most outrageous, rebellious thing I could do. Which has absolutely nothing to do with why I'm pursuing motherhood. But it's an interesting part of this experience. As much as I'd love my kid to have a relationship with his or her grandfather, I will not ever allow my child to have a bond with someone who would make me (and potentially that child) feel shame. Especially shame about where that child comes from. I fear my father would not accept a child that was born from a sperm donor. Particularly one whose sperm I handled personally in a public restroom.

I hope he proves me wrong and can love and accept a grandchild regardless of their origin story. But I don't—I can't—build my life around what he thinks anymore.

Chapter Five
Paging Dr. Patronizing

I N 1884, A PHILADELPHIA PHYSICIAN named William Pancoast altered the history of fertility medicine when he orchestrated a pageant, of sorts, to assist a couple struggling with infertility.

Without informing the couple—a thirty-one-year-old woman and her forty-one-year-old merchant husband who had been rendered infertile by a bout of gonorrhea—he polled his medical students to determine which among them everyone believed was the most attractive. Then, Pancoast coordinated to have the winning student produce a sample on a day when the woman came in for a procedure. As a handful of his students looked on, Pancoast anesthetized the woman with chloroform and inseminated her with the sperm using a rubber syringe followed by a pack of gauze shoved against her cervix.

The woman became pregnant and later had a healthy baby boy, at which point Pancoast informed the husband—but not the wife—of the deceit. The men agreed that she was better off not knowing the truth of her impregnation and the child's paternity.

This deception became the first successful, recorded artificial insemination using donor sperm in US history, and began a pattern of secrecy, lies, and taboos that have long surrounded donor conception in the United States.

The story of Dr. Pancoast's deception only became public in 1909 when one of the medical students who witnessed the insemination published a letter disclosing the entire procedure in *Medical World* journal. Before the letter was published, the student, Dr. Addison Davis Hard, revealed the truth to the AI offspring, by then an adult.

Ultimately, Pancoast was just one of many barbaric doctors in the nineteenth century during the rise of modern Western medicine. Medical history and research have long failed to prioritize the needs of all patients, particularly women, racial and ethnic minorities, and the LGBTQ+ community. Reproductive medicine has a long history of exploitation.

Decades after Pancoast's success, modern medicine is still trying to address the problem of infertility, so I don't know why I thought it would all be easy for me.

I HAD BEEN SO CERTAIN that all it would take was a little bit of sperm to make my belly swell, my menses dry up, and life to come forth from my body. Yet, month after month, my womb failed to provide fertile soil for the donor sperm I had been introducing to it at perfectly timed intervals.

I shouldn't have been surprised. Before I even met The Conquistador, I went to a fertility doctor to check my hormone levels and egg reserve (a predictor for how many eggs you produce). The news was grim. It was not likely that I would get pregnant easily. Still, I didn't believe what the doctor told me. He wanted to move straight to expensive treatments, while I wanted to do intrauterine insemination (IUI) in the clinic with a known donor. Going through a clinic was my preference because it felt more legit than home insemination, and I had good fertility coverage. But my doctor balked.

"Oh no," he said. "You need to go through a bank."

"Why? I'll have the sperm donor do STI, genetic, and sperm analysis testing."

"Because I have thirty-four years of experience. I know what I'm doing."

"Um, but, is that just your policy, or . . . ?"

"It's the law. The FDA requires it."

"But I know people have used a known sperm donor in clinic settings before. I'm not crazy."

"Well, sure. But they have to go through a very specific, FDA-approved process."

He explained that the sperm donor would need to be tested for all diseases, and then he would only have a one-week window during which he could provide samples—though samples must be produced at least two days apart, so seemingly only two or three vials of sperm could be produced. If I needed more, I would need to shell out for another round of testing during a new one-week window. Then, the donor's sperm would need to be frozen and quarantined for six months, after which the donor and the sperm would be retested for all diseases. If the donor was clear, at that point I could use any surviving sperm to attempt IUI. When I tried to calculate the cost of the entire process, it would have roughly added at least an extra $6,000 per two or three vials of sperm obtained.

The donor would also be required to undergo a psych exam (at my out-of-pocket cost), as would I—regardless of where I got my sperm. This was a mandate that was not thrust upon married couples, which seems gross and biased. But no one asked me.

"That's ridiculous," I told the doctor. "Surely there must be clinics that waive this quarantine process. It's my body. I'm an adult. I could theoretically go sleep with whoever I want to get pregnant. I should be able to decide whether I feel safe using a person's sperm after standard testing."

"There isn't a reputable clinic that will do it any other way," the doctor said, smugly.

It turns out he was lying, or at the very least just plain wrong. I later learned that other clinics do, in fact, allow people to waive the six-month quarantine, and some even allow fresh sperm to be used for IUI and IVF—as long as the donor is what the FDA defines as a sexually intimate partner. The problem is that the FDA's definition is unclear, and many clinics simply classify a sexually intimate partner as anyone whose sperm has been inside the patient's body—even through artificial insemination. By that logic, a patient at the clinic should be able to use the sperm donor for IUI or IVF—without jumping through the hoops posed by the FDA. I was not far enough in my journey to know this, however.

With a bit of uneasiness, I realized at that point that I was going to have to do home insemination, after all. Obviously,

The Conquistador and I soon after pursued the NI path, but it would have been nice to have the option to go through a clinic without thousands of dollars of unnecessary costs and a massive delay—particularly now that my doctor had made my reproductive system sound like a broken vending machine in desperate need of a good shake and constant replenishment.

Now, with The Lawyer, I was personally handling the sperm instead of leaning on the familiar comfort of the medical system. No sterile clinics or metal stirrups for me.

I have to say, The Lawyer was incredibly reliable. Like clockwork. It didn't matter what the holiday or what was going on in his life, he always came through with three fresh donations, three days in a row, each cycle. Signing a mortgage on a new house? He'll make it work. The weekend he was moving? Not a problem. Christmas Day? Big deal.

I had heard so many horror stories from so many women about donors who flaked out or demanded sex, it was hard to believe I had gotten so lucky. This was a truly good and generous man who was helping me, for free, out of the kindness of his heart. He was literally getting nothing out of it beyond the satisfaction of helping someone and knowing that his DNA would carry on—and that any resulting child would be in good hands.

But after several months of working with The Lawyer and getting zero success, I was tracking my cycle meticulously and it was becoming apparent that something was wrong. The average twenty-eight-day cycle is broken down into two main phases—the follicular phase and the luteal phase, with ovulation occurring in between. My luteal phase—the ten-to-sixteen-day window after you ovulate—was too short, ranging from six to nine days. When that happens, any potential embryo doesn't have enough time to implant in the uterus before menstruation starts, washing any chance of a baby away.

I went back to Dr. Patronizing and begged him to prescribe me medication to extend my luteal phase by staving off my period.

"I know exactly what's wrong," I explained. "I've been tracking my cycle, and timing everything perfectly. I just get my period too early. Everything I've read indicates that adding progesterone to my routine after ovulation could help delay my period long enough for embryo implantation."

He didn't even look me in the eye as he answered, dismissively: "Oh no, I couldn't do that. Not while you're doing home insemination."

"I don't understand. Why not? I'm not asking you to inseminate me. Just give me a fighting chance the way you would if I was married and trying to do this."

"I have thirty-four years of experience. The answer is no."

I was desperate. Dr. Patronizing's answer was tantamount to patting me on the head.

In the end, I did something dishonest. I waited two days, called back the doctor's office, and asked to talk to the nurse.

"Good news! My donor and I decided to be in a relationship. We're going to be a family!"

"That's wonderful!" the nurse chirped.

"So, I was hoping to come in so I can get a prescription for progesterone?"

That was all it took. I still find it hard to believe that a simple, artless lie made the costly red tape immediately disappear. They didn't just give me a prescription for progesterone—they cheerfully started me on monitored coitus cycles, which meant they would have me come in almost daily leading up to my ovulation and give me letrozole, a medication designed to boost the growth of my follicles (the sacs that contain the eggs), giving me the best possible shot at getting as many mature eggs as possible. I also had a trigger shot, which induced ovulation at the perfect time, when Dr. Patronizing informed me that my eggs were ripe and thus it was the appropriate time. After ovulation, they gave me progesterone to hold off menstruation as long as necessary for implantation.

In reality, my "boyfriend," The Lawyer, and I were inseminating at specific times suggested by the doctor—who thought we were a couple having sex at those times. Of course, I asked my donor's permission to engage in this lie, as it could have legal implications later on, should I seek child support from him (which I wouldn't).

I never got a reasonable, clear answer from my doctor— beyond his repeated proclamations about having thirty-four years of experience—explaining why he wouldn't help me pursue motherhood with a donor who could actually have some connection to the child. I tried to explain the amount of research I had done, the better psychological outcomes for children who have the opportunity to know more about their donors, but he wouldn't budge or elaborate on his reasoning. It felt like he enjoyed having control.

THE THING ABOUT INFERTILITY IS that it is utterly dull, yet completely all-consuming: Tracking my temperature, charting my cycle and dates of ovulation, taking eighteen different supplements. I had long since quit smoking, cut out most of my drinking, and was going to acupuncture. I didn't even microwave food in plastic anymore because I was worried toxins could leach into my food and harm my fertility.

I was tired of being in my own brain. All I could think about was having a baby, where I was in my cycle, and how my cervical fluid was looking.

Checking cervical fluid—sometimes called cervical mucus (ew, let's all agree not to call it that anymore?)—is a way of judging where a woman is in her cycle. Women typically have some vaginal discharge most days of the month. Early in the cycle this discharge tends to be dry and sticky, then by days seven through nine it becomes creamier in texture. By days ten to twelve it thins out and becomes wet and clear, until around days thirteen and fourteen, when it's runny, like the texture of egg whites—that's the good stuff. It's that egg-white fluid that protects the sperm from the otherwise inhospitable environment of the vagina, and helps it coast along, providing a smooth path toward the cervix.

Each day I would get up around seven a.m. and take about twelve different supplements that were designed to improve fertility via various means before going on a four- or five-mile walk.

I read about these supplements in Rebecca Fett's *It Starts with the Egg*, a book that covers lifestyle changes women can make to improve their egg quality. I was spending more than $400 a month to keep up with it all.

- A prenatal vitamin with folate—a more effective form of folic acid that prevents neural tube defects

- CoQ10, also known as Ubiquinol—a supplement that can help improve egg quality

- Vitamin D—insufficient D can contribute to infertility

- Alpha-lipoic acid—believed to promote cycle regularity and the egg's ability to mature and fertilize, as well as embryo development

- Vitamin E—helps with cellular repair and believed to help prevent the most negative effects of premature aging

- Vitamin C—improves hormone levels and helps with luteal phase defect

- N-acetylcysteine—said to improve ovarian response to the fertility drugs I was taking to boost the size and maturity of my eggs

- Omega-3—believed to help with conception

- Magnesium—controls the follicle-stimulating hormone that stimulates the ovaries

- Glutathione and cysteine—supports egg quality by maintaining metabolic balance

- PQQ (pyrroloquinoline quinone)—shown to stimulate the growth of mitochondria

- NAD+ with Resveratrol—higher levels of this coenzyme is correlated with better egg quality

I had to be careful not to take all my supplements on an empty stomach; I had vomited a few times during my morning walks because I couldn't tolerate them without a little food.

In addition to the supplement routine, several times a day I would pee on a stick, which would let me know when my lutenizing hormone was present. This would appear (like a pregnancy test) as two pink lines on a little strip of cardboard. When I hit my peak—and the two lines were as dark as can be—it meant that I was about to ovulate; in other words, my eggs were about to drop out of my ovaries and start making their way down the fallopian tubes. Once this happens, the sperm have twenty-four hours to get to the egg and fertilize. For that reason, most recipients are encouraged to inseminate leading up to the actual day of ovulation, because fresh sperm can live up to five days in a woman's body, but once the egg is absorbed into the uterine wall, it's too late.

I used my free time to scroll through the Facebook fertility groups to look for other women who fit my profile (age thirty-nine, low egg reserve, and looking to become a single mother by choice). I clung to the happy stories of success and tried to dismiss the repeated heartbreaks I saw posted day after day. Despite what my doctor said, I was certain that I wouldn't be one of them, especially now that I was getting medicated assistance with my home inseminations. If and when I did get pregnant, being over thirty-five would make it—in medical terms—a geriatric pregnancy. I shudder at this terminology but couldn't dispute it.

The odds of a woman being infertile start at around 7 percent in the early twenties and rise to 15 percent in the early thirties. After thirty-five, the likelihood rises to more than 20 percent and reaches nearly 30 percent by age forty.

I was going into the clinic several times a month for the doctor to monitor how many eggs I was producing each cycle and how big they were getting so the clinic could advise me on when to inject a "trigger" shot to spur ovulation. But even with that assistance it was becoming hard to ignore the void in my womb. Women over thirty-five are considered infertile after six months of trying. I had gone through eight medicated cycles.

The entire process was so exhausting, and I couldn't think about anything else. I was becoming a boring conversationalist. I sensed my friends were cringing every time I provided another incremental update on my journey, whether it was discussing my discomfort with the monthly trigger injections, my frustration with Dr. Patronizing, or just the constant yearning for a child. I struggled to discuss anything other than getting pregnant.

As a woman this was the one thing that I was supposed to be able to do. I had taken birth control pills for fifteen years to prevent this very thing from happening, in fact. And now I was holding regular cocktail parties in my uterus with all these medications and supplements, yet I had nothing to show for it.

My quiet confidence in my body and this journey we were on together started to waver. Little by little, I was folding into myself like a sad, crumpled origami crane that just realized it would never be able to fly. I bargained, I denied my reality, and I grieved what I thought the world owed me: I wasn't getting pregnant. I was most probably infertile. My world became gray and dreary and getting out of bed became impossible. The worst part was that I had no one to share this with. No partner in my grief, no comforting arms to hold me, and no mouth to kiss away my tears and whisper that they, too, hurt in this exact same way.

Women everywhere have struggled with infertility. But it's a special kind of loneliness when you have no one to share it with beyond awkward overshares with coworkers and gut-wrenching exchanges with old friends over the phone.

I would lie awake at night with my hands palm-down on my stomach. I meditated, rhythmically repeating to myself: "I am the mother; I am the child." I'm not sure how that mantra came to me, but it felt so natural to honor my own inner child and the child I was trying to welcome. The words just fell out of my mouth one day. I didn't have a partner to support me through this time. But I did have a collection of incredible female friends who supported and fortified me as I discovered and navigated my infertility challenges.

In addition to the many wonderful women who I already had in my life, I found a Facebook group for single moms by choice in the greater D.C.-Maryland-Virginia region. The group included many women who were already moms, and they would organize playdates and girls' nights and all the things I dreamed of being a part of when I had my own little one. But I also noticed several women who still considered themselves "thinkers" (they hadn't fully decided whether to pursue solo parenthood) and "triers" (women actively going through fertility treatments to get pregnant). I made a post catering to the latter two, asking if anyone wanted to start a group chat and maybe get together to discuss where we were in our journeys.

The response was huge. Before too long, we had a large group chat going, and I quickly organized the first get-together at my place—it was still the midst of the pandemic and the huge outdoor space in my backyard was ideal for a socially responsible event where we could be seated in a circle, six feet apart from each other. I looked around at these women, all intelligent, hardworking professionals who hadn't found love and partnership yet refused to give up on their dreams of motherhood. The core group was established that day: eight of us who would stick together and share our victories and tragedies on this journey. I was the only one pursuing the freelance sperm route. At first, I sensed the others felt I was a bit odd for following this path. They gave me some wide-eyed stares initially, but as I shared more details and explained my rationale and all the testing my donor had gone through, they all seemed to "get it"—even if it wasn't a choice they would have made. For these women—most women—the unregulated online sperm market is still too much of a wild card to pursue. Plus, it admittedly comes with additional work (vetting) and frustrations (flaky donors) that can be completely avoided by going to a sperm bank.

This group is where I met Karen Sullivan, who is forty-three at the time of this writing. Karen has curly brown hair, a wide, infectious smile, and a year-round tan thanks to her love of hiking and all things outdoors. An environmental economist with the Environmental Protection Agency, she has a grit and resilience that was forged during a childhood in which she learned to persevere in difficult circumstances. A child of divorce, she had to cope from a young age with her mother's bipolar disorder, and her father later committed suicide. I only learned these details after years of friendship; Karen is not a complainer and does not waste time feeling sorry for herself.

We first connected when she was forty and her fertility journey was technically just getting under way. She had already had a bumpy start after attempting to check her fertility and freeze her eggs at age thirty-seven.

The doctors took her blood, tracked her cycle, and quickly told her then that there was no point, as her egg reserve was so low that she was far better off immediately trying to get pregnant. As one would expect, Karen was devastated. She thought it wasn't unreasonable to freeze her eggs at her age, figuring she was being smart and still had a shot at buying some time before motherhood was off the table.

Karen had a ton of student loan debt and wasn't financially ready to have a child on her own. For three years she worked hard and took on extra hours and side jobs to pay down as much of it as possible and establish some financial stability.

When I met her, at age forty, she was fresh from her first few IUIs (intrauterine insemination—when the doctor uses a long tube, or syringe, that travels through the cervix into the uterus and deposits washed donor sperm inside at precisely the right time). The doctor had told her that she had such a low egg reserve that her chances of success from IUI and IVF were about the same. She had spent some months comparing donors at sperm banks until she settled on one, and had her first insemination in May 2020. It didn't take. The very next IUI did work, however—and for a fleeting moment she was filled with euphoria.

Then she started bleeding just before her six-week scan and lost the baby.

She did four more IUIs before giving up and realizing it was time to move on to IVF. As a federal employee, Karen's insurance didn't cover this procedure, and she didn't have $20,000 to $30,000 sitting around for this purpose. But then she found CNY, an Upstate New York clinic whose mission is to make fertility treatment more affordable. For about $4,000 (plus travel and accommodation costs) Karen was able to start the process with them in the summer of 2021.

Karen was certain that shelling out a ton of money for IVF would be a sure thing, but during her first two attempts, she didn't respond to IVF at all. Doctors told her to consider donor eggs because hers were too old and too unhealthy to produce a baby. Another doctor recommended trying to lower her medication dosage to see if that would work. This approach, known as mini-IVF, is based on the theory that some older women may "overbake" their eggs when taking max doses of hormones that stimulate the ovaries. The idea is that lower doses can more gently spur the natural process of egg development in these women.

Using that approach, Karen went through two more rounds to get one day-three embryo. In the early days of IVF, this is when embryos were transferred. These days it's preferred that the embryos get to five days, known as the blastocyst stage, before transfer. But women who struggle to respond to IVF will often freeze and transfer the three-day embryo because there's less risk that the embryo will arrest and stop developing in the petri dish.

At one point, doctors in Virginia found that Karen had one large, healthy-looking egg in her ovaries. At her doctor's advice she drove up to Albany, New York, in a snowstorm to have the one egg retrieved and fertilized. Unfortunately, she had already ovulated by the time she arrived. It was a wasted trip, and nothing could be done.

By now, Karen was starting to lose hope. But even though her doctors suggested she use donor eggs, she persevered with her own eggs and got another day-three embryo. Karen went on to do one more round of egg retrievals, having them extract one egg from her and then use two donor eggs. Doctors fertilized all three, but only the donor eggs took.

Karen transferred her two day-three embryos made with her own eggs but was unsuccessful getting pregnant. She took some time to reflect and "wrap my head around" using the embryos she had made from the donor eggs.

I've always been struck by how strong and stoic Karen is. She is not one to talk about the heartache of infertility, even though she's walked one of the hardest paths of all the women in our group.

Karen is always traveling, taking little weekend adventure trips and visiting friends in other parts of the country. During her time going through IVF, she had to back-burner traveling entirely—a weighty sacrifice for my worldly friend.

Karen and I also shared the grief you must dwell in before you can move past the life you thought you'd have and embrace becoming a solo parent.

"I always pictured that I'd have a baby with a husband," she said. "I will miss that piece of it. But I will also have control. I won't have to make decisions with a partner, which could also be good. There's positives and negatives to either side. And I think I just try to focus on the positive side."

I agreed with Karen here. I don't want to have to negotiate things like how to discipline a child, whether they should attend public or private school, or—God forbid—fight to get them vaccinated. While it is easier to have another person around, being the sole "decider" has a certain appeal.

Karen and I both have heard from our married friends with children that their husbands don't help them anyway. But those women do have to negotiate day-to-day difficult stuff like: Who's going to pick up the kid? Can they stay out overnight at a friend's house? Do they really need to eat all their vegetables?

"Every little thing, you've got to be on the same page, or you've got to have a discussion and figure it out," Karen said. "Seems much easier to just figure it out yourself."

Karen has been there for me through some of my lowest moments on my own fertility journey. When I've mentioned dark moments in our group chat, she's taken the time to reach out to me directly and make sure that I'm okay, that I don't feel alone. This natural nurturing quality practically oozes out of her pores: the way she always wordlessly is the first to help the host clean up at our wannabe-mommy gatherings; how she knows just the right moment to pitch in to help the women who are now moms chase their little ones around; the way she can get babies and little kids to laugh with her.

Like most women who struggle with infertility, we both wasted energy wishing we could go back in time and check our fertility earlier. But there's no way to win the game of what-ifs.

My irrepressible friend does have some disappointment and resentment toward the medical industry. Women in their twenties and early thirties are not encouraged to know where their fertility stands. And while media is full of stories of celebrities and social media influencers getting pregnant at increasingly older ages, those stories fail to cover things like Karen's six-year journey to-date.

"In our culture, as women, we're not really told anything about this when we're in our ripe, prime fertility years, when we're in our twenties. No one really ever said anything to me like 'Oh, you want kids someday? Well, you should think about freezing your eggs.' No one ever mentioned anything related to that. Even in my thirties, doctors asked me, did I want to have kids? I'd say yes, and then that would be the end of the discussion with my general practitioner. As if there was nothing more to say."

Karen's thoughts resonated with me. I spent so much time chowing down birth control and fearing pregnancy, it had never occurred to me that I could have the opposite problem. Why are doctors being gatekeepers to our ability to realize our dreams of motherhood? And I'm not just talking about the paternalistic approach of those like Dr. Patronizing. Where were my primary care physicians and gynecologists when my fertility was slipping away?

In the meantime, Karen's persistence appears to have paid off: She is currently fifteen weeks pregnant with a girl she conceived with a donor egg and donor sperm. She's been doing lots of reading and picking out baby books that help explain donor conception, because she wants to be able to tell her daughter—from birth—where she comes from.

Paging Dr. Patronizing

After so many miscarriages and tens of thousands of dollars spent on failed pregnancy attempts, Karen has been cautious about allowing herself to hope. But passing that fifteen-week mark and learning that her prenatal testing (NIPT) came back normal was a turning point for her.

"I'm starting to believe it's really going to happen," she told me, a few hours after announcing her pregnancy to her family.

She's taken some time to work through her disappointment about not having a biological child, and for the moment is in a good place.

"This really can happen," she added, her voice almost dreamy. "I can become a mom. I'm really hopeful now. More so than ever."

Chapter Six
Don't Call Them Diblings

F OR MUCH OF HER LIFE, Sarah Blythe Shapiro knew her biological father as #314.

To the sperm bank, he was a number rather than a name.
Along with some basic self-reported facts about his ancestry,
this was all the information Sarah had about her biological
dad. However, it was enough of a foundation for the curly-
haired twenty-three-year-old Yale graduate student to imagine her father. While most children read picture books before
bed, Sarah, at the age of four, sometimes read her biological
father's donor profile, trying to glean some sort of significant
and telling information that would make her feel closer to the
dad she'd never met.

"I think subconsciously, I just projected a lot onto this person, because I wanted him to be what he couldn't be. And I had a
lot of really toxic male figures in my life. And so he just became
invincible practically," Sarah said.

Whether it was her thin frame, dark skin, fast speech pattern, or talent for music and singing—she was choir director
for HaZamir: The International Jewish Teen Choir, among

others—Sarah wondered, obsessively, about which traits may have come from her bio dad.

The New York City native grew up mostly in Chicago, raised by a single mother by choice, and despite its being a loving, positive relationship, Sarah always acutely felt the absence of a father figure. When she was finally able to start the process of meeting her mother's sperm donor, at age eighteen, she soon discovered the reality was excruciatingly far from what her imagination had promised.

Most people who use sperm banks likely don't realize the difficult and lengthy process involved when an eighteen-year-old decides they want to meet their donor. It's not uncommon for donors to decline contact, sometimes because they've already met with so many offspring that they are overwhelmed and too exhausted to take on any more relationships.

The industry could do a better job at making sure that men know what they are getting into and are better prepared for the reality that future children might wish to seek a relationship with them. Sperm banks could also support the passage of proposed state laws that would set strict limits on how many children each donor can produce.

Currently, sperm banks say they self-regulate so that any one donor doesn't overproduce. But it seems impossible for them to get an accurate count, because many recipients never report pregnancies or births.

Most banks now offer open ID at age eighteen as an alternative to total anonymity, meaning the donor has only consented to the disclosure of his identity when the child turns eighteen. It does not guarantee any new information, let alone a meeting, beyond that disclosure, and sometimes a donor has no interest in meeting or developing a relationship with their off-spring. Donor-conceived people often say they never asked to be here, and are sick of being told they should just be grateful they're alive. They feel they deserve what many of us had the fortune to experience: a relationship with both biological parents.

As soon as she turned eighteen, Sarah started by reaching out to the sperm bank and asking for a meeting with the donor. It took several deflating months before she heard anything back from him. She was disappointed to learn from the sperm bank that he wanted to stay anonymous and would only communicate with her through a bank mediator or a blocked number. The mediation carried on for months, during which Sarah knew him only as "C"—not a big step forward from the three digits that she had clung to for most of her life. Every time she felt their conversation was making progress, she would ask for more. And he would retreat.

"It was really, really, really hard going back and forth like that, because I had all these questions. And he felt like I was being pushy," she said.

More than a decade before Sarah was conceived, the Iranian American experimental filmmaker Caveh Zahedi was still in film school in Los Angeles. It was 1986 or 1987, and Caveh had just started the graduate program at UCLA when he spotted a sign on campus: WANTED: SPERM DONORS.

It seemed like a painless way to make extra cash, and the clinic had a facility near his daily classes, so it was just a matter of stopping by before or after school and ejaculating into a cup. He received $35 per deposit, with a max of three donations per week, or $400 per month—easy money.

The donating stopped when the bank eventually told him they didn't need his sperm anymore because they had enough to meet the level of demand for his product.

"I assumed that meant there had been no requests and they didn't want to waste their money on me," Caveh said, genuinely thinking he hadn't produced any children based on how abruptly he was dismissed from the donation process.

He was wrong. Sarah was one of the children produced from his sperm, and she's identified fourteen additional half-siblings since she learned Caveh was her donor in 2020.

Caveh says he has no idea if there are more children beyond those whom Sarah has found—the sperm bank never provided him with any numbers, as is typical. The idea of meeting any of his children from donation makes him nervous since he's a semi-public person and worries that they're initiating contact because of a desire for financial gain.

Sarah had no interest in Caveh's money, but her excavation into her biological father's life soon got uncomfortable, for both of them.

She learned that Caveh was in active sex addiction for ten years before entering recovery, though he never disclosed that on the donor forms. He also never reported having Crohn's

Disease, which Sarah has, as does her grandmother on her mother's side.

The hardest part was feeling rejected by Caveh—whose name she had actually discovered on her own with a little bit of sleuthing (she knew he was an Iranian American filmmaker who taught at a New York City university, and put the rest together).

"He was very, very cold for a long time," she said. "He's still cold. It's not the greatest relationship. He doesn't like how pushy and forward I am. But I think his idea of being pushy or forward is simply insisting on my human rights and deserving this information. He doesn't like my style of going about it. But I think he's a dick. It's a whole thing."

Caveh says he felt kindly toward her, but didn't want to be responsible for her emotional well-being.

"Then I got this letter from her that was touching, and a little scary in that it seemed like she was having very big expectations that I didn't think I could fulfill or wanted to fulfill, to have some kind of father figure in her life," he said.

He tried to be nice, but not too nice. Caveh was concerned because Sarah's note seemed to indicate that she was expecting a lot from him. He was willing to give her certain information about her genetic background but found himself withholding any emotional connection. Sarah wanted a father figure in her life. But: "In my mind, I didn't sign up for that."

Caveh says he was profoundly conflicted when Sarah came swooping into his life. He wanted to know more about her, but to do so would risk leading her on. He feared giving her the false impression that he could be there for her in the way that she craved.

"I could tell this was a person with a father-sized hole in her heart and she had projected a lot onto me as this idealized, mythical figure who was waiting to embrace her," Caveh says. "She seemed like a little girl who really wanted her father's approval. It was scary. I could just tell there was something here that was a little bit off, or too much."

Caveh says there were turning points that made him feel closer to Sarah and helped him see that the genetic connection they had was real.

"She sent me some videos of her singing original compositions, and it was really good," he said. "She was clearly an impressive, intelligent, artistic person. And I think that, more than anything, convinced me to go along with this thing, whatever it was."

Their first in-person meeting was unorthodox, to say the least. Caveh traveled to Chicago for a new showing of one of his productions with his filmmaker friends. He asked her for permission to film their first interaction—before he had even provided her with his actual identity.

"I felt really violated," Sarah said. "I was like, 'Why don't you get to know who I am, and I can get to know who you are?' But eventually, he admitted to me who he was. And I agreed, because honestly, I wanted it to be filmed. I felt like, 'I've been so wronged in this whole situation that I want a chance to be famous. And I want a chance to have this documented. I want to be able to remember this and have people filming it.'"

Caveh has somewhat of a cult following. It was easy for him to call on a bunch of his fans to bring their camera equipment and shoot the entire first meeting, which lasted for three hours.

When Sarah first met Caveh, she immediately noticed similarities. Like her, Caveh has a slight build and speaks in rapid-fire bursts. But she didn't share his affinity for cannabis or his—at times—cruelly direct way of speaking to others.

The Washington, D.C.–born child of Iranian immigrants has cobbled together a bizarre IMDb profile featuring works in a genre that could best be defined as hyperconfessional. The *New York Times* described one of his most recent creations, *The Show About the Show,* as having an "abject, self-defeating, ethically questionable, maddeningly original approach to documentary." The show is literally about the making of the show and each episode rehashes the episode before it. (I tried to watch it and it was painful.) Caveh seizes on the moments that make the people in his life feel humiliated and uncomfortable. The filmmaker has won awards for his work; he also has children of his own.

At one point during their first meeting, Caveh offered Sarah a hit from his bong. When she graciously declined, Caveh asked her if she cared that he smoked. Sarah told him it wasn't a problem.

"He just sat there smoking in front of me," Sarah said. "I was like, 'This is so weird,' because it's so different from my own upbringing. My mom would never do that."

Sarah was struck by the man's neuroses, and just how much he was nothing like the strong, loving image she had constructed in her imagination.

"He was worried that I was going to judge him. I didn't judge him for his decisions and his past. I judged him for how he went about his relationship with me and for some of the unkind things he said."

At one point during the filming, he said to Sarah: "I'm not even sure if I like you."

Sarah paused as she recalled this before raising her voice to retort: "I am your daughter!"

Since that meeting, Sarah has been trying to cope with the fact that her biological father, with whom she shares large brown eyes and a talent for Ping-Pong, is a major disappointment.

"I think he's a sociopath," she said. "I think he has narcissistic personality disorder. He cannot stay in a marriage. He was a sex addict. He lied about his ethnicity. He is so strange."

The effects of his eighteen-year absence, combined with their bizarre first meeting, ricocheted across Sarah's personal life over the next several years following their unsettling meeting, coloring most of her interactions with men. Her vivid self-awareness was not enough to stop her from creating a pattern of unhealthy, self-destructive behavior.

Sarah cycled through many unhealthy relationships with toxic men, which she views as a direct reaction to her craving for the father figure of her dreams.

"It was so traumatic. I would kind of cling to all these boys like, 'Where's my dad, where's my dad, where's my dad?' And at one point, one of them rejected me and said, 'I don't really like you, you're coming on too strong and pushing for clarity.'"

Caveh had also told her that—the same day that a guy said those exact words to Sarah. It destroyed her.

Sarah is angry at her biological father and at the sperm bank. She's since reached out to other siblings she found through genetic testing sites Ancestry.com and 23andMe, as well as the Donor Sibling Registry, a site designed for people born from sperm bank donors to find each other. She let them know the identity of the sperm donor so they won't have to go through the monthslong, arm's-length screening process that she did.

She was angry when Caveh told her that the sperm bank had given him a free therapy session to help him cope with the fallout of being a donor. Sarah was not extended the same offer, stating that the bank prioritizes donors above the children they create.

Sarah believes that every child has a right to know their biological parents, including any biological siblings, from the start. She thinks the only ethical way to have a child with a donor is to introduce them to the donor at birth and always leave the door to contact open. No waiting for an eighteenth birthday.

Hearing this made me a little uncomfortable because I was working with The Lawyer, who obviously wasn't willing to meet the child from birth. Instead of turning away from Sarah's pain, I tried to sit with that discomfort and examine it. Did I need to change my own course?

Don't Call Them Diblings

The controversy of Sarah's opinion quickly becomes apparent if you raise these issues in the sperm donation Facebook groups. Potential parents don't want to hear that they could be harming their future child through secrecy and by denying them access to their donor. Many recipients don't ever want to see the donor again after they become pregnant. And the anonymous donors don't like the implication that they owe anything to their offspring.

A Belgian study examining sperm donor motivations and attitudes found that 46 percent of candidates wanted information on how many children would be conceived using their sperm. Eighty-two percent of the participants were willing to provide basic—but anonymous—information about themselves to offspring. Just 26 percent said they would still donate if their identity was eventually revealed to the child.

Similarly, a Danish study found that half of the participants would no longer donate if they couldn't be guaranteed anonymity, and only 17 percent said they were certain they would follow through with donating without anonymity.

Sarah believes the sperm bank industry needs to make a radical change to abolish anonymous donation and make it possible for the donor-conceived to know their biological parent from birth. She views this issue as an up-and-coming human rights issue. Sarah maintains that she's not trying to hurt anyone's feelings—but parents of donor-conceived children can't predict or control how their kid will feel about his or her conception and biological connections. Why shouldn't the donor-conceived be entitled to something akin to the open adoption approach that is so often encouraged these days?

Lesbian couples in particular have said that it feels like a heteronormative slap in the face to hear that their child needs a link to their biological father. It can become very tense, very quickly on the Facebook pages when this topic comes up. Understandably, the non-gestational parent doesn't want to feel that they are less than, or not enough, for the child.

But I found Sarah's lived experience a more compelling argument. I was moved when she spoke about how her pain had grown into a festering wound that infected every corner of her life.

Caveh says he still struggles to understand Sarah, and felt like she rebuffed his efforts to get to know her. His way of doing so was by including Sarah in producing a film that he felt she lost interest in. He also wanted to play music together—he'd offered to break out his recorder and do some duets with her over video chat. Caveh called her, but Sarah didn't return the calls. He felt his biological daughter was rejecting him, even though he didn't particularly feel the drive to cultivate a relationship with her.

Caveh was relieved when she started pulling away.

More often than not, the stories of donor-conceived people are marked by deception. Many DCPs are lied to their entire lives about their biological history and feel betrayed and devastated by parents who keep their biology a secret. Others are told the truth, but due to anonymity required by sperm banks can grow up feeling profoundly aware of the absence of a father.

Often, donor-conceived people feel pressured to put their parents' feelings first—for example, by showing little or no outward interest in meeting a biological parent, often despite an acute desire to pursue such a connection. It becomes a sort of role reversal in which the child is taking care of the parents' emotional well-being, says Melissa Lindsey, founder and executive director of Donor Conceived Community, a nonprofit support group.

"It puts strain on the relationship," says Melissa, who is donor-conceived. "And it prevents closeness because there's a feeling of needing to hide and I don't think a person can hide their life and have it not affect the rest of the relationship."

These feelings become most acute at moments in life where one is supposed to feel a closeness with their family, such as sitting around the table for a holiday dinner.

This disconnection that many donor-conceived people feel often compels them to connect with biological siblings. Many use spreadsheets or binders to keep track of these new, sprawling extended families, regardless of whether that's five or fifty people. But these relationships are often complicated and filled with anxiety because it's difficult to know others' boundaries—how much contact each person is willing to have, and whether they want to know details about the donor.

Some only want to know medical updates about siblings and the donor, while others want to know about siblings but nothing about the donor. Others only want to know if someone dies. Some want meaningful relationships with their donor, or however many half-siblings they can find. There's a whole spectrum of lived experiences and emotions that donor-conceived people go through, Melissa says.

"THE TERM 'DIBLING,' I DON'T know if you've heard it?" Sarah asked. The annoyance in her voice was unmistakable.

"Dibling" is a word created and used by recipient parents to talk about their children's donor-conceived siblings from other families. Sarah and other donor-conceived people often prefer to be called siblings, half-siblings, or donor-conceived siblings. Sarah has thirteen half-siblings, though not all were willing to meet.

Sarah says the term minimizes the connection donor-conceived people can have with their biological siblings. She believes recipient parents use the term because it makes them feel more comfortable, rather than putting the comfort of the donor-conceived first.

"I know that I didn't grow up with them," Sarah says. "But that doesn't change the fact that we're related."

The first half-sibling Sarah discovered was living in Utrecht, in the Netherlands. That person never responded to outreach Sarah sent via the sperm bank, and, for years, was the only biological link she could find. Eventually, however, she got a notification on the sibling registry website about another sibling, a woman who was ten years older than her.

The first time this half-sibling reached out was "mind-blowing" for Sarah. As an only child, it meant so much to her to connect—for the first time in her life—with someone who shared a biological connection via Caveh. They never met in person but periodically call and exchange emails.

Sarah has attempted to make contact with all thirteen siblings and has been successful hearing back from many.

The second sibling Sarah found was a woman her own age (who declined further contact); this sibling had a twin brother named AJ whom Sarah has since had the chance to meet in person.

Sarah recounted story after story of deceit within her own extended genetic family. In one case, the husband and wife who used the same donor as Sarah's mom were going through a divorce after never having revealed the truth to their children. The nonbiological dad who raised the children told them about their half-sister (Sarah) to spite his wife, who didn't want the children to know they were donor-conceived. The children were young, around seven and eleven, and didn't want to meet Sarah. Who can blame them, when their very existence was suddenly at the center of a familial implosion?

"It's just not easy to uphold relationships with this many people," Sarah says. "It's just exhausting, emotionally. You can't do it."

There were other stories, too.

Another of Sarah's siblings had her donor-conceived origin hidden from her for her entire life—until her nonbiological father died and her mom revealed the truth. Similarly, AJ and his sister didn't find out about being conceived by donor egg and sperm until they were preparing to leave for college.

Even before Sarah met AJ, she was struck by his voice on the phone. It sounded remarkably like her own.

Then, the first time they met, Sarah says it was as if she recognized him on some subconscious level. They looked enough alike that there was an instant, uncanny familiarity. Sarah observed that they shared a fine-boned build, darker complexions, and the same curly hair.

They immediately found a comfortable rhythm after meeting up at UCLA's Hammer Museum, an arts and cultural center known for its contemporary collection and progressive exhibitions and public programs.

As the siblings explored the different exhibits together, they unpacked everything they knew about their genetic father and his family, talking through all the weird moments Sarah had with him. For the first time in her life, she had someone—a brother—with whom to share her donor-conceived reality. Later, they headed out to get ramen for lunch and to play Ping-Pong—something that Caveh had claimed to be good at on his donor profile.

"It was so surreal yet really natural," Sarah said, noting that they realized they had similar tastes in romantic partners as well.

Twenty-two-year-old AJ was the third half-sibling that Sarah connected with through Ancestry.com. She first spoke with his twin sister before linking up with AJ and forging the beginnings of a real sibling bond. AJ and Caveh have an uncanny resemblance—that slight frame, delicate facial structure, and olive skin. They share the same wide, brown eyes and slightly prominent nose, with an overall impish, magnetic quality.

AJ learned from Sarah that Caveh was the donor at the beginning of his sophomore year of college.

"Sarah was very good at sleuthing and digging to find information," he said. "She asked if I wanted to see the yearbook picture of the sperm donor because she thought that I looked like him."

Sarah sent AJ the photo. He was overwhelmed because he never thought there could be a stranger out in the world who would look so much like him.

But AJ decided he doesn't want to meet Caveh, feeling like Sarah's experience was enough of an answer for him about that side of his biology.

He softened, however, when discussing the idea of eventually meeting his egg donor, his voice bright with vulnerability and hope. While the correspondence with his biological mother has been through the mother who raised him, everyone seems open to communicating. But his mom has been slow to respond to her egg donor.

"I think a little bit of it is that she's just uncomfortable with me needing this other parental-type figure. Or she just has a lot on her plate. I don't really know. Once I'm antsy enough, or once I feel like I have enough free time, then I probably will ask to meet with her. It's obviously a little awkward. The stakes still feel very high. But I would like to meet her."

AJ grew up with a mother and father, and never experienced the same acute sense of parental absence that Sarah described.

He was raised in Los Angeles, and his parents were older by the time they decided to have children. Fertility was an issue, so the couple opted for double donors—sperm and eggs—and became pregnant via IVF. Neither AJ nor his twin sister had any idea about their conception until just before they left for college. Their mother sat them down and took a very serious, concerning tone, her voice dropping several octaves. This worried AJ. He had no idea what to expect as she danced around the topic before finally blurting out the truth about their biological parentage.

"My first thought was 'Oh, that's kind of big.' And then immediately after I thought, 'But this shouldn't be very big'—at least for my relationship with my mom," AJ says. "She seemed nervous about how we would react. So I made sure to not react too much."

Despite everything, AJ says his origin story hasn't made a big impact on his life. He understands why his parents kept it a secret for so long; they admitted that they didn't know the right thing to do. At the time they became pregnant, there weren't as many answers about how to handle these situations. They were also afraid that the twins would see them as less of their parents—which AJ says is absurd.

AJ is still figuring out what all of this means for himself, beyond his relationship with his parents. He says he's adapted to his new reality so well because he had a great home life and two parents.

"I've always known who my dad is, he's always been my dad. I never felt like there was anything missing for me," he says. "I assume that Sarah feels more strongly because it's all been such an obvious part of her life where there's a hole."

In 1917, Dr. Frank Davis, an Oklahoma physician focused on treating infertility, was one of the first to go on the record linking artificial insemination to eugenic goals, meaning he believed medicine should approach human reproduction with the goal of increasing the occurrence of desirable heritable characteristics. This ideology has historically been linked with racial bias, particularly after it was adopted by the Nazis during World War II.

Davis was the former superintendent of the Oklahoma Institution for the Feeble Minded. His experience in that role led him to the belief that intellectually disabled and mentally ill people should be confined and cured. Conversely, those with superior genetic traits should focus their energy on reproducing and spreading their desirable qualities to as many spawn as possible.

He was genuinely worried about "race suicide," which was how he described the declining birth rate in Christian countries. In addition to performing surgery on women, Davis also performed artificial insemination and taught couples how to perform the technique on their own at home. He claimed his efforts cured "many cases of barrenness."

Soon after, experimentation with artificial insemination started to take off, with a 1928 survey of medical literature from around the globe yielding 185 reported instances of artificial insemination, with 65 resulting in successful live births.

The decade following that study saw a massive boom in artificial insemination, and by 1941, AI was responsible for ten thousand live births.

Around the same time, the British doctor Mary Barton was being criticized internationally for publishing a report on her efforts with donor insemination in the *British Medical Journal.* Unlike many of the men in her field at the time, Barton understood that male infertility was just as common as female infertility. Her sperm donor solution to help childless couples was controversial; the idea of heterosexual couples raising children that were not biologically linked to the father made people uncomfortable. Some experts speculate this goes back to the evolutionary benefit for infants who look like their fathers—males of many species are more likely to stay and help the family unit survive if they believe the child is their own. It could also be because most societies focus on patrilineal descent. It was eventually revealed that Barton used her husband's sperm to produce as many as six hundred babies through her practice.

In the 1950s, an estimated twenty thousand children were born in the US via AI. In 1953, two doctors in Iowa produced the first successful pregnancies using frozen sperm—a critical discovery in terms of monetizing sperm donation. The birth of three resulting babies in 1954 led to the formation of the first-ever sperm bank out of a University of Iowa clinic. At the time, the *Cedar Rapids Gazette* ran the headline "Fatherhood After Death Has Now Been Proven Possible."

A survey of physicians who were likely to perform artificial insemination, conducted in 1977, found that 379, or 80 percent, of the 471 respondents were, in fact, using donor sperm for AI. This accounted for 3,576 births that year. Most doctors chose the donor for the recipient, and typically they found the sperm donors at local universities. The donors were only screened for a handful of genetic diseases, if at all, and were largely chosen based on how similar they looked to the husband of the recipient.

Single women accounted for just 10 percent of those on whom doctors had performed the procedure. In these early days, women were typically inseminated twice per menstrual cycle. Donors were frequently changed from one cycle to the next, with only 17 percent of doctors being used consistently.

A third of the doctors said they had used multiple donors on the same woman in the same cycle—making it that much harder to determine the child's true paternity. At the time, sperm donors' identities were never revealed for legal, privacy, and societal reasons.

The first baby born from in vitro fertilization (IVF) was in 1978, in England. The first born in the US was in 1981, following a process that required the mother to drive twenty minutes to a hospital for fertility drug injections three times a day. (The procedure has evolved over the years and now most women inject themselves or get help from a partner.) The resulting American child, Elizabeth Carr, is now in her forties and has advocated for making IVF and fertility treatment more affordable.

The first commercial sperm banks also opened in the 1970s, eventually leading to the so-called Nobel Prize Sperm Bank, or the Repository for Germinal Choice, which was established to collect the sperm of the world's best and brightest and then spread that high-value seed to spawn geniuses across all the land, apparently.

The inherently controversial Escondido, California, bank was in operation for twenty years, eventually closing its doors in 1999. Its founder, multimillionaire Robert Graham, was a fan of eugenics, which was a popular concept among white supremacists and Nazis.

Graham publicized his plan to fill the world with genetically "superior" children, spurring widespread outrage and pushback—but not before he had collected sperm from three Nobel laureates. After widespread public pressure, two of the laureates withdrew permission to use their sperm—to this day their identities are unknown.

The third and only remaining laureate donor was William Shockley, a white supremacist and fan of Hitler's own eugenics attempts. When that was discovered, even *Saturday Night Live* took a stab at mocking the Nobel Prize Sperm Bank, with a skit entitled "Dr. Shockley's House of Sperm."

Some have attempted to find out how many children were produced by the bank (Graham eventually extended his search for donors beyond just Nobel laureates), with the journalist David Plotz concluding in his 2001 book *The Genius Factory* that 217 children were conceived and born because of donations from the bank.

From the beginning, secrecy, or deception, was the point. Sperm donation started out in the shadows, carrying a shame that loomed large for the people and couples who had to turn to that option due to infertility. Many donor-conceived people were lied to and denied the truth about their origins. Those who learned of their parentage generally had no way of knowing who their biological father was.

SPERM BANKS HAVE GUIDELINES THEY must follow related to testing, procedures, and storage. But in the US, they have never been regulated in terms of how many offspring they will allow any one given donor to produce. The American Society for Reproductive Medicine has guidelines that call for a limit of twenty-five live births per donor, per population area of 800,000, but there's no way to enforce that. Plus, not all recipients report their pregnancies and live births, so it's easy for that guideline to be surpassed without the banks realizing it.

Part of the problem is that Americans are loath to have to report their pregnancy to banks or a donor-conceived registry—

it's just too invasive, too Big Brother for us. So, no such law has been passed in the US. There's also no registry of donors, so it's easy for them to go from bank to bank.

Meanwhile, strict limits are enforced in other countries and jurisdictions, including the UK, where each donor is limited to helping ten families. Many states in Australia have laws that place limits on recipient families, often requiring a donor's sperm to no longer be used after five to ten families have been helped. Australia does import sperm from other countries to address the shortages that these limitations create. However, imported donor sperm has often already been used to procreate widely in the country of origin, meaning each child created could still have dozens of siblings internationally.

Compounding the problem with lack of oversight on how many offspring can be produced by one donor, US banks have historically shared donors with each other through partnership networks that allow a donor to have his product available from multiple banks around the world under the same donor number. This can make tracking the number of live births per donor more challenging.

There are also sperm consignment programs, in which banks provide sperm to be stored directly at fertility clinics. Recipients who go this route can get cheaper sperm, but they have fewer options to choose from and the sperm is often older and from inactive donors (so you may not get more vials for siblings in the future). This also makes it tougher to track or limit any one donor's production. Seattle Sperm Bank even vaguely references its consignment program on its website and in its donor agreement.

Donor-conceived people say banks know they are failing at self-regulating donor limits, and that failure is obvious, given the many different groups of siblings who realized— after finding each other on consumer genealogy websites— that their parents obtained the sperm of the same donor from multiple banks around the country, or even overseas.

While it's possible that one donor may donate to several banks, DCPs say that the situation is so widespread that banks must still be allowing proliferation and distribution of sperm from donors who likely reached or surpassed limits.

Donor-conceived people have been getting organized, as evidenced by the formation of the US Donor Conceived Council (USDCC) in 2021. This nonprofit, volunteer-run advocacy group is funded through private donations, primarily from donor-conceived people and lesbian and gay parents. The group represents the growing movement of donor-conceived people who want their voices heard in state and local government. The organization has the goal of pushing the assisted reproductive industry to make changes that would ensure the needs of donor-conceived children are met.

They face an inherent challenge, however: They are ultimately pushing for laws that will primarily affect the lives of people who haven't yet been born. And in a post–*Roe v. Wade* era, some are fearful that could be seized on by the anti-abortion movement as seeking to establish rights for the unborn.

The group's leadership fiercely disputes the notion that its work in any way represents the interests of or establishes rights for the unborn. USDCC leadership says they're committed to only drafting and supporting legislation that strikes any language referencing the unborn.

The industry agreed to meet with USDCC and other stake-holders to hear concerns of DCPs in a first-of-its-kind meeting in Los Angeles in October 2022. Multiple sperm banks and egg banks took part, as did RESOLVE: The National Infertility Association, along with industry professionals, mental health experts, lawyers, and academics. Topics included the potential for real limits on donor family units, the importance of maintaining historic medical records, and the need for identity of donors to be released at eighteen.

However, the industry resisted meaningful change, warning that further legislation around these issues could lead to higher prices for consumers—which could in turn drive more people to the unregulated sperm market.

In the first six months of its existence, USDCC helped push through the Donor-Conceived Persons and Families of Donor-Conceived Persons Protection Act in Colorado. The bill, which is the first of its kind, bans anonymous sperm or egg donation in the state. Sperm banks cannot provide anonymous sperm to recipients from Colorado—even if they travel to another state. Sperm and egg donors in that state must agree to have their identity released to their donor-conceived offspring when the child reaches age eighteen.

In addition, the law requires all sperm and egg donors to consent to having their medical history released when any of their donor-conceived offspring turn eighteen. The responsibility of gathering and regularly updating each donor's medical information falls on the shoulders of the sperm bank or agency that collected the gametes in the first place. It also gives parents of the donor-conceived person the right to obtain non-identifying medical records on the donor.

The bill also placed a twenty-five-family limit on the total number of recipient families that can be made with a given donor's sperm. That's consistent with what some banks say they are already doing. For example, Fairfax Cryobank advertises its family limits as twenty-five in the US and fifteen abroad—again, USDCC disputes that those limits are currently enforceable or accurately documented.

Even with those limitations, a recipient parent must understand that their donor will be allowed to produce children for a total of forty family units, says Jamie Spiers, a donor-conceived person and advisor to USDCC.

If each family has two children, that's eighty children from one donor.

The family limit issue is very important to USDCC, as many donor-conceived people struggle to maintain relationships with all their siblings.

Unlike sperm donors, the Colorado law limits egg donors from undergoing more than six egg donation retrieval procedures—unless the egg donor is known at the time of donation. However, an egg donor in her twenties could produce potentially dozens of healthy eggs during each cycle.

The Colorado law also mandates education: prospective parents must be informed about the potential harm of family secrecy around conception, and that their donor-conceived children will have the legal right to know the donor's identity.

Similar bills recently failed in Maryland and California, making Colorado the lone outlier that has made progress on this issue. Jamie declined to comment on whether USDCC had plans to pursue new legislation in additional states, saying the group is meeting with various state lawmakers and assessing dynamics in different parts of the country as they develop a plan for the 2024 state legislative sessions.

Opponents to this kind of legislation are concerned the bill could have unintended consequences—for example, some sperm banks may find it too costly to comply with the law's requirements and could just stop offering their services in that state. Colorado only has one sperm bank, and that one will no longer be able to compete in the anonymous sperm donation market, which could hurt their bottom line.

Another worry is that the limits on how many children a donor can produce would hurt sperm banks financially—which often only accept a very small percentage of the men who pursue sperm donation in a clinic setting. They would have to charge more per vial of sperm, they say, because they wouldn't be able to make as much money off of each donor. This is a serious concern because the steep cost of sperm and assisted reproduction already counts out many families.

California Cryobank has actually created a "donor reserve" program, in which aspiring parents can pay $70,000 for the Platinum program to have a sperm donor exclusively to themselves, with supplemental vials included. The Silver Reserve program limits the number of family units a donor can produce to two to ten for the price of $35,000 per family and an additional $3,000 per vial of sperm. This is a clear indication that sperm banks have been profiting from the customer demand and are trying to maintain their bottom line by attaching a higher price tag to limiting family units. It is also clear that sperm banks have historically had a financial incentive to get as many children as possible out of each donor. Many banks are rethinking this in the current climate, but they are businesses, and the pressure to remain profitable is very real.

CINDY SPIERS FEELS MISLED AND deceived by a sperm bank that she believes put profit before the best interest of her own children and others conceived with the same donor.

Cryogenic Laboratories, Inc., which has since been absorbed by Fairfax Cryobank, is one of the nation's largest banks. Cindy has a receipt showing that she spent more than $15,000 in 1995 to purchase seventy-five vials of the donor's sperm to allegedly buy out the last of his supply. Cryogenic Laboratories had told her fewer than five other families had successfully used the same donor. Cindy wanted to spare her daughter Jamie and her children from having dozens of siblings.

However, the bank called the donor back the very next year and asked him to provide more sperm—allegedly only for siblings of existing children in the two families. But extensive records and the existence of younger and younger siblings indicate that the donor's sperm was used to continue donating up until at least seventeen years ago.

According to the donor, when the bank called him in 1996, they indicated that the new donations were purely for families that had already successfully had a pregnancy.

That 1996 round of donations was the last time the donor provided sperm to the bank. He was stunned when he found out how long his DNA continued to be available to produce more children.

Jamie Spiers has thirty-seven half-siblings that she knows of, ranging in age from sixteen to thirty-one, found through genealogy websites, the Donor Sibling Registry, and independent investigation. After much careful calculation, Cindy and Jamie estimate that the banks distributed roughly 1,700 of the donor's vials.

"The notion that banks were potentially sharing resources didn't occur to me," Cindy says. "It wasn't a global mindset in 1995. I had no concept that they were swapping sperm."

Cindy and Jamie believe multiple banks share vials with each other through affiliated networks. The bank took Cindy's money even though they must have known the donor's sperm was still being provided to families around the country and would continue to be used indefinitely.

Cindy loves Jamie to pieces but could never have imagined how much she would regret choosing an anonymous donor to build her family. Cindy chose anonymity because she worried that her child's biological father might pursue custody at some point down the line. She had read about child custody cases from the 1980s and 1990s of lesbian mothers losing their children to their heterosexual biological fathers and Cindy, who is gay, didn't want to take any risks.

From a very young age, Jamie knew that she wanted to one day meet her biological father, though Cindy was afraid of what could happen if she did.

"I set us up for failure by trying so hard to lock down my little family," she says.

"My mother started disclosing about my conception when I was under the age of three," Jamie says. "She used the 'body parts' narrative. She explained that it takes boy parts and girl parts to make a baby and that she went to the store and bought the boy parts that she needed."

This was a narrative that persisted throughout most of Jamie's childhood. Cindy had worked hard to divorce the donor as a person from the gametes she had purchased.

Jamie is thin—almost frail-looking—and her pale, freckled face and long, wavy brown hair belie her twenty-six years. She oozes youth while simultaneously carrying herself with an air of authority. Her speech is direct, each word plucked from her mind after careful consideration, and uttered with a deliberate, quiet intensity. She let her mom know early on that she wanted to know who her donor was, maybe even meet him.

In her late teen years, Jamie developed what she calls a "maladaptive behavior" of calling men who matched the sperm donor's description and asking if they had ever donated sperm.

"Most of them hung up on me, logically," she says.

The disagreement drove a wedge between mother and daughter. They have since repaired the relationship, but Cindy still struggles with the decision she made to use an anonymous donor. She tears up easily when discussing her regret.

Cindy can understand why some people choose anonymity and why those in the world of unregulated sperm donation may seek to not even actually know a donor's full name—they're operating from the same place of fear. Now, she realizes, that fear was unfounded. Her daughter's desire to meet her donor didn't have anything to do with the amount of love Jamie has for Cindy.

Jamie's relationship with her mother has grown deeper and more open since Cindy started accepting and even embracing her daughter's mission to connect with her sperm donor.

"It's only within the past few years that we have been able to discuss this, and she has changed her views," Jamie says, noting that her mother was haunted by the unknown.

Another critical reason Jamie and Cindy would have liked to be able to contact the donor early on was because Jamie had hereditary health issues that she would have been more prepared for had she known about them. Mother and daughter tell me the bank failed to maintain current records revealing the health issues—even after the donor reported to them that his sister had died of the same thing Jamie was diagnosed with. The US Donor Conceived Council wants to require banks to continue to maintain medical records on donors, even after they go out of business.

In addition to the guilt Cindy felt over her decision to use an anonymous donor, like many parents she admitted that she was shocked when her child didn't turn out along the lines of a miniature clone. As a result, it was difficult, at times, for mother and daughter to understand each other. Jamie was direct and blunt, different from her mother, who as an attorney has a more poetic, or diplomatic, delivery. Jamie finally got answers when she ultimately met the sperm donor and saw that so many traits—including those that had made her so different from her mother—were mirrored by her biological father.

"She's a mini him," Cindy says of Jamie and the donor.

Cindy had specifically sought out a smart person with a math background. Jamie and her other children all share that strength.

"They're like aliens to me," Cindy says.

Finally meeting her donor was a major turning point in Jamie's life. But it didn't happen overnight.

From the age of twelve, she was searching her donor's file to figure out his identity. She thought she had a decent chance of finding him. He had been in a unique PhD program—which was how she managed to figure out the school he attended by the time she was fourteen.

"This is also when I started researching the bank's practices," Jamie says. "I was able to narrow it down by ruling out other PhD programs after learning that the donors were mainly local to the cryobank's location at the time he donated."

Once DNA tests became more popular, she was able to combine genealogy records online with public information from the PhD program to get his identity. She took the information she could find in the donor's file and created a family tree on a wall in her apartment. Jamie took the closest DNA matches she could find to the donor and built out a family tree based on each relative's publicly available trees. She then expanded the tree until she connected to a name that was not in the records from the PhD program. After some additional research, she was able to find name change documents that connected the tree to the donor, who had legally changed his name prior to publishing his research during the PhD program.

She kept her distance for years but found comfort in knowing who he was. Other half-siblings followed the same trail of breadcrumbs, she later learned. Jamie and some of her half-siblings came up with the nickname of "Mr. DNA" for the donor as an inside joke.

Mr. DNA tells Jamie that he never anticipated so many children would be produced with his sperm.

Jamie has been in contact with her biological father for a year, though she determined his identity six years prior.

Last year, Mr. DNA accidentally sent a friend request to one of Jamie's half-brothers while trying to switch between viewing different Facebook profiles of his various donor offspring. The half-brother who received the request immediately contacted Jamie, and they wrote a message to Mr. DNA together. It took him a little while to notice the message, but Mr. DNA was happy to connect.

Thanks to the Donor Sibling Registry, "Mr. DNA was able to find our social media and watch us from a distance for many years," Jamie says. The donor had known about seventeen of the thirty-seven offspring by the time Jamie contacted him.

The accident that brought Jamie and Mr. DNA into each other's lives couldn't have had a happier ending. They have forged a meaningful bond, a connection that has helped Jamie better understand who she is and where she comes from.

Mr. DNA said, via email, that meeting Jamie has been "a rich and rewarding experience."

"I'm always pleasantly surprised by our many similarities, such as extreme curiosity," he said.

Over time, he's changed how he feels about anonymous sperm donation, and has learned a lot from Jamie about how it can affect the people conceived in darkness.

"Jamie and the other people that I helped create have grown into adulthood and given voice to their experiences," Mr.

DNA wrote. "They have expressed their need, and desire, to better understand themselves through knowing their origins, accessing my evolving medical history, knowing their siblings, learning about traits shared with me, and even interacting with me."

He said the world has changed dramatically since he donated and that it's time for the industry to adapt appropriately.

"It seems that the only option is to adjust to the change and recognize the reality of the situation," he said. "Finding out you are donor-conceived is probably really hard, but that you have forty siblings must be pretty mind-blowing. I have empathy for donor-conceived individuals."

Chapter Seven
Designer Babies

IN THE ERA OF INSTAGRAM and the all-important pregnancy photoshoot—typically followed by newborn and mommy-and-me photoshoots, and then monthly photo updates for the entire first year of a child's life—people in modern America spend a lot of time thinking about their baby's public image.

This emphasis on appearance and the perceived social status that comes from getting lots of "likes" seems to draw some recipients to the unregulated sperm market as a way to pursue some notion of a designer baby. Some women in the Facebook groups have such a fully formed image of their future child that it seems they might be disappointed if the kiddo popped out without the precise features they envisioned.

For example, some recipients request only certain types of Black hair, or specific nose shapes. I've seen some recipients insist they don't want a donor with ancestors from certain countries in Africa because those ethnicities have, in the eyes of these women, undesirable facial features. Additionally, some Black women have specifically sought out white or Asian donors, in some cases due to a desire to have a lighter-skinned or half-Asian, half-Black baby.

This apparent desire, by some recipients, to choose a donor based on a very specific combination of ethnicities and facial features is inevitable. People do this on sperm bank websites, too—selecting a donor based on a certain ethnicity, or eye- and hair-color combination. The blue- or green-eyed light-skinned Black donor is a popular request on the Facebook pages.

Sometimes recipients are merely looking for donors that look like their partner who is unable to produce sperm (either because it's another gay woman, a trans man, or an infertile man). But often, these requests seem driven by a desire to pick out the physical features they want to see (or avoid) in their child.

Another aspect of this is the white women who are seeking to have a non-white baby due to a desire to further racial equity in America. I have no objections to interracial relationships or donation—but it does sit wrong when I see women fetishizing the idea of having a mixed-race baby as if it provides them with some kind of social cachet, and without contemplating the responsibility of preparing a child to be non-white in America or connecting them with their cultural background.

"It is a red flag," says Latrice, an African American woman who has an eighteen-month-old baby with her wife, thanks to Ron's assistance.

"It's actually quite annoying and frustrating to see white women seeking Black donors in that way," she says. "It is a completely different ball game raising Black kids in America. There should be some level of experience with the Black community when you decide to bring a biracial baby into the mix, because some of those conversations are really tough to have and you don't necessarily have them with your son or daughter as a white woman or a white man."

Jennifer, a white single mother by choice with two daughters, says that while she initially didn't want to factor in race when choosing a sperm donor, ultimately she had to be honest with herself about her capacity for raising a non-white child.

"The white liberal woman in me was like, 'Oh, race doesn't matter, any donor will do.' And then I realized, no, there are so few donors of color out there for people who need or who want that. It would be unfair for me to take that option away from someone else. I'm white, and like many white women, my immediate circle is not that diverse. I live in Pennsylvania, which is not that diverse. I have no business trying to raise a multiracial child. So, my first criteria was that the donor had to be white."

IN THE UNREGULATED SPERM MARKETPLACE—unlike the sperm banks—donors make the decisions about which recipients to help, and which to ignore. This often means that many donors, particularly the discerning ones, will steer clear of recipients who seem to emphasize their designer baby goals more than their overarching desire to become parents.

It also means that some donors may avoid working with certain recipients for the wrong reasons.

When Monique and her wife set out to find a sperm donor on the Facebook pages, she could tell that attracting the best candidates would be competitive. The thirty-eight-year-old homemaker took time to draft a thoughtful request, explaining that she and her wife were educated, financially stable, and ready—emotionally and otherwise—for a baby. She included a photo of the couple, hit "post," and waited. And waited.

That first effort didn't get a single comment or result in even one direct message expressing interest in helping the couple.

"The white recipients did get more replies just based on the comments on their posts," said Monique, who is African American. That was true even when the white recipients posted minimal information about themselves. Those who shared sexy selfies and little else would get dozens of comments from eager donors.

Ultimately, the unregulated sperm market is a microcosm of the real world—it has the same racism and biases. Despite that, many women of color enter the world of freelance sperm because they feel they aren't being served well by the medical profession when it comes to their fertility and reproductive health. Others are frustrated by the shortage of Black donors at sperm banks—which account for only 1 to 4 percent of all donors at the nation's four largest sperm banks. About 4 to 6 percent are Asian. For some, this is reason enough to seek out freelance sperm donors.

"It suggests that you're not the intended audience; you're not the intended recipient of this treatment," says Camisha Russell, an associate professor of philosophy at the University of Oregon, and the author of *The Assisted Reproduction of Race*, which evaluates ideas around race in assisted reproductive technologies.

Another issue was that Monique felt that white donors seemed to sexualize her and fetishize her as a Black woman.

"They want the big butt, or it just seems like Black women are sought after on the groups for sexual reasons, not because they're a good person with the right qualifications to be a mom," Monique says. "Whenever I would get a white donor that would reach out to me specifically, they always wanted partial or natural insemination. They just wanted sex. It was never like, 'I want to help you out.' It was 'Will you send a picture of yourself?'"

Monique is not alone. Other recipients of color say they felt passed over by donors based on their race or ethnicity.

"It's weird," says recipient Rose Marie, a moderator in the Facebook groups who used Ari Nagel as a donor. "Do I want you to just be honest, and say you don't want to be my donor because you don't want a Black woman? Or do I want you to just say, 'Oh, I'm not interested at this time.' I can't say for sure that donors have rejected me based on a racial thing. But sometimes it comes across that way."

I also talked to many Black women who said they didn't feel race was an issue at all in the groups—they were just tired of men pressuring them for sex, in general.

However, one NI-only donor named Jonah, who is white, told me that he rarely donates to Black women because he objects to the grammar of their posts and is concerned that, in his opinion, they often appear to have a lower income, and therefore are more likely to pursue child support. He also described recipient posts in which "their profile picture is them smoking a joint and giving the middle finger. It's obviously going to be one hundred percent no, you know?

"Not that I'm racist or anything, but I've tended to find that a lot of African American recipients, a lot of them, they just don't complete, like, full sentences," Jonah said. "Or they just act real, real trashy. I get that impression from a lot of them. They don't really have, like, a sturdy background financially and that knowledge is one of my big concerns."

This blatantly racist attitude validates the stories from Black women in the community who say racist undercurrents could be why they struggle to find decent donors.

Often, the plight of Black women struggling with infertility is not viewed as a real problem in society, or even in fertility clinics, Camisha says.

"An infertile Black woman doesn't keep with stereotypes about women of color, which are that they are these excessively fertile people who are going to be on welfare," she says.

There's a legacy of distrust of medicine among marginalized communities, Camisha attests. That's true in reproductive medicine, and largely due to a long history of abuses by the medical community, including forced sterilizations and coercive uses of long-acting contraceptives.

Systemic racism in medicine goes back a long way in US history. J. Marion Sims was dubbed the "Father of Gynecology" in the mid-1800s for developing surgical methods to treat the female reproductive system, and for inventing the speculum. But his true legacy was the cruelty he wielded in the name of medical progress: He achieved all his medical breakthroughs by performing surgeries on enslaved women without their consent or anesthesia.

The problems continued into the twentieth century, as evidenced by a 1973 lawsuit that revealed that more than 100,000 poor—and predominately Black, Latina, and Indigenous women—had been subjected to forced sterilization. This occurred between 1907 and 1932, a period during which thirty-two states established laws allowing the government to sterilize women who had been labeled insane, feebleminded, or otherwise unable to care for themselves.

Most of these laws have been repealed, though a version of the law remains on the books in my home state of Washington.

"People don't think that the world needs more Black children," Russell says.

In other words, medical history and research have long failed to take into consideration the needs of all patients, particularly women, racial and ethnic minorities, and the LGBTQ+ community. Often fertility clinics, doctors, and even sperm banks act as gatekeepers that can determine whether someone receives care and what that looks like.

"African American women experience an atrocious amount of bias or prejudices in medical settings," says Alexis S., an African American recipient in the freelance sperm world who asked that I use only her first name and last initial. Alexis has an illuminating smile, and jokes about being an antisocial hippie. She works for a commercial cleaning company and is studying a trade that she's confident will provide a decent life for her future child.

Alexis is asexual and aromantic, meaning she isn't interested in sexual or romantic relationships. She wants to be a single mother by choice and found her way to this world due to the high cost at sperm banks and her disappointment in the medical profession's attitude toward Black women.

"I feel like Black women often get the 'tough' or 'strong' labels put onto us, and because of that, whenever we are in a medical setting trying to describe our symptoms, we are not immediately believed," she adds. "There have been numerous times where I have gone to the ER for severe pain and other symptoms only to leave feeling like I was never heard the entire time. This is why it took sixteen years for me to be diagnosed with stage four endometriosis and fibroids. Those experiences have left a permanent bad taste in my mouth, and I am reluctant to seek medical treatment. I am also worried about how I will be treated as a SMBC in medical settings. I know that I will probably get endless amounts of questions regarding 'who the father is,' and while annoying, I am prepared to proudly state that I am the only parent by choice."

Monique says she finds racist donors annoying more than anything and tries not to dwell on biases and stereotypes that have long been part of her life. She persevered in the online world and connected with Ron, the donor who only does AI to keep his addiction in check.

"I chose Ron because he asked me the important questions first, which is something that you don't normally see," she says. "They're usually asking, 'What questions do you have for me?' And so, I liked it when Ron asked me, 'What do you do? How is your health?' He vetted me to make sure I was a good recipient."

Ron asked tough questions. He wanted to know why Monique wanted to have a child; what kind of mother would she be; what could she and her wife give the child?

"Then, when I met with him, he just was very sincere on insisting he didn't want anything extra. He wants to see that the kids are growing up healthy. He likes it when I share the kid's pictures on Facebook. He just wanted to help and wanted to make sure that his DNA would be carried on and taken care of."

For Sarah's entire life, she had discreetly clung to the "whiteness" of being able to say she was a quarter French, a detail she gleaned from Caveh's sperm donor profile when she was just a little girl.

That turned out to be a lie.

"I didn't really think anybody would want me if I was just Iranian," Caveh said. "I was trying to get the job, but both my parents are Iranian, and I remember thinking, 'I'm probably not going to get hired if I say that.' Since my mom was a bit of a Francophile, I just said French on one side."

Sarah felt confused when she discovered this new layer of deceit. The donor's background was the reason she had studied the French language throughout her schooling. She had a "huge" problem with the way Caveh devalued their Iranian bloodline, even though it mirrored her own biases.

"I'm horrified, completely furious," she said. "For a long time, I had all this internal racism about being a Jew and being Iranian, and the only redeeming quality I could find within my race was being French, because it was more 'white.' I grew up in a very white environment. So, realizing I wasn't French forced me to realize that I am a person of color. That kind of took me down a whole spiral of delving deeper into my own ethnicity, my own history."

She was most upset by the fact that Caveh never thought to correct this information with the cryobank in the thirty-three years since he had donated.

Caveh apologized. And he still says he feels terrible about what he did.

"I was embarrassed about lying," Caveh said.

AJ had his own struggles with the race and ethnicity question related to his egg and sperm donors, because he had grown up with white Jewish parents who were—as far as he knew—his biological mother and father.

"I've always looked pretty racially ambiguous," he says. "For a very long time, ever since I could remember, I've had people asking me, 'What am I?' And so of course, I asked my parents when I was little, and my mom is German and Romanian, Ashkenazi Jewish, and my dad didn't actually know his father. So, there was always kind of an X factor there that could just explain away anything that wasn't explained in terms of how I looked."

AJ's father would always say that his own father was from southern Spain—a fact AJ saw as an explanation for his darker complexion.

"I grew up never thinking about it too strongly. Because I could tell that they were always a little ambiguous in their answers, which makes a lot of sense now."

When he finally took a 23andMe test after learning he was donor-conceived, AJ said he initially got the wrong information. His test showed him as 50 percent Iranian and 40 percent generally Asian (a combination of Indian, Mongolian, Chinese, Korean, Indonesian, and Malaysian).

"It was wild to me, because I had never considered I could be Asian," AJ says. "I was going into college, and that's supposed to be a very unique time to explore your identity. And, in the interest of that, I joined the Asian American–Pacific Islander mentorship program at my school. Now, looking back, there was something a little wrong with that, like, I definitely did not look Asian, not even mixed, but I don't know, I saw those results. DNA is supposed to be accurate."

Months later he was telling an Indian friend about his results, and she was skeptical. He pulled up 23andMe to show her the proof, and—to his shock—the results had changed. Now it showed him as 50 percent Iranian, 10 percent Anatolian (the ethnicity of a people who live in the westernmost peninsula on the continent of Asia), and 40 percent Central Asian, which is because the egg donor is Uzbek.

"So, not at all East Asian in any way, which was the club I participated in all my freshman year," AJ continues. "I look back at that and it feels so odd. All the interactions that I had with people at the time, saying, 'Oh yeah, I know I don't look Asian, but I deserve to be in this space, too' . . . I didn't know. God. That's been pretty difficult to grapple with, and kind of funny. Also, kind of embarrassing."

Knowing his identity has sent him afloat a bit. He's not just "white" anymore, but he's not an easily checked box on most forms, either.

"In America, most kinds of census-type racial breakdowns don't really have categories that account for that. It's definitely led me to do a lot of soul searching about, like, whiteness and race in America and about how much race is a social construct and how much of it is just the culture that you've been inundated with and how much it is just how people treat you and what they think you are."

All of this has led him to the conclusion that he identifies as Jewish, more than anything else.

"That's the culture that I grew up with," AJ says. "That's the food that I know. I went to the Jewish day school. I learned Hebrew, I can read Hebrew. I was bar mitzvahed. It's such a distinct culture that I'm totally a part of, and it isn't reliant on changing 23andMe tabs."

Chapter Eight
The Kids Are Going to Be (Mostly) Fine

I NERVOUSLY TYPED OUT THE text message, deleted it a few times, started over, and finally came up with this:

> Hey, Babes! I miss you, how are you? I know this is going to sound crazy, but I've been trying to get pregnant for months now. I want to be a single mother by choice, and have actually been working with a sperm donor here in D.C. But it occurs to me . . . you would be an excellent candidate for the role of biological father to my baby . . . Would you ever consider being a sperm donor? We could have a contract outlining that I would have full custody, and you would never be required to pay child support. It really would mean a lot to me for my child to have a relationship with the donor. And I know you're someone who will be in my life forever. No pressure. Please let me know your thoughts. I'm happy to answer any questions you may have. xoxox

I gulped and hit "send."

I had known David for fifteen years. It had been at least six months since we'd spoken, so while he was used to getting lengthy texts from me out of nowhere, this was something else entirely. As a gay man, his path to parenthood was never going to necessarily be a straight line, but I wasn't sure how he felt about having a child or helping create one. I had been inspired to take a hard exit from the Facebook pages and was legit kicking myself for not thinking of calling on David sooner. He had all the shallow and the important qualities that any recipient could want: He's a dashingly handsome American boy, of Jewish and French heritage, from upstate New York. He's tall (six feet three), with dark brown hair, deep-set brown eyes, and a devilish grin. David's sharp-witted and sarcastic as hell, but an absolute teddy bear with the people he loves. He can be a tough guy and use his imposing stature when he wants to—usually when his protective mode is activated on behalf of his female friends.

David is also highly emotionally intelligent. He's incredible at reading a room, observing different people's temperaments and picking up on when anyone may feel low or left out—and he makes a concerted effort to make them feel included, or to put a smile on their face. Being in David's orbit feels comforting, like being pulled to safety by a gentle, centrifugal force.

My stomach flip-flopped. I paced around my kitchen and cracked my knuckles as I awaited his response.

I didn't have to wait long. My phone chimed with the *donk donk* sound from *Law & Order*, notifying me I had a new message. David had responded:

FUCK YES!!!

Now it was my heart doing the flip-flopping. I couldn't believe he said yes—not just yes, but he didn't even have any further questions. This was the David I knew and loved. We could go months or even years without talking, but I could reach out to him out of the blue and he would be by my side to support me in a heartbeat.

Over the next few hours, we talked about what level of involvement he would have with the child (as much as he wants—which we both expected to amount to between one to six visits per year). I explained what I and the kid would need from him (a willingness to be available to answer medical or family history questions—or periodic curiosity inquiries from the kiddo). I envisioned him as a fun uncle type of relative, who would also be a good male role model for my child. He would love my kid and be open and honest about being the biological father from day one.

I couldn't believe it. I had found a detour around my predicament, and now had a donor who would be an incredible asset in my child's life. I immediately started making plans to travel to Boston, where David lives, for my next insemination.

I have a note-to-self recording I made (I occasionally made these brief journal-like recordings at different points along my journey) while I was in the air on my way to see him:

"This is Valerie. It is December twenty-six. I am on an airplane right now. About twenty-five minutes outside of Boston. I'm on my way there to meet my friend David. And will immediately begin demanding that he produces a sample so I may inseminate! This is a really big adventure. I'm a little nervous that it won't work. Because I don't know that the timing is perfect with my ovulation, but there still should be a chance, so fingers crossed. I'm nervous about making this commitment to doing this with my friend. I don't want anything to jeopardize the friendship because it's very precious to me. Most of all, I'm just very hopeful. I really hope it works and that I can become a mom."

It was absolutely freezing cold in the city on a hill when I arrived. David was housesitting for a friend in an adorable brownstone that was fully decked out with a tree, lights, and decorations for Christmas. As soon as we got settled in the house (following a proper bear hug, David had changed into his big blue bathrobe, and I was sporting my pandemic uniform of yoga pants and a sweatshirt—no bra), we plopped onto the big, overstuffed couch so I could spill my guts about everything I had been doing on my motherhood journey. I could always just relax, be myself, be real, with David.

Initially we had a bit of a gush session about how much we loved each other. We hadn't seen each other since I moved to D.C. from New York. When I lived in Brooklyn it was easier for him to come see me, and our shared passion for music often had us going to concerts together, including Radiohead, the Yeah Yeah Yeahs, and the Pixies.

This was a very different kind of quality time.

"I love that you're going to bring a child into the world who will be brought up with openness and kindness and also intelligence," David said. "I know you would put your all into anything you can do for a child. That's why I was comfortable with doing this."

He squeezed my hand and gave me a reassuring smile.

I was reminded of when we first met in Albany, New York. I was covering state politics for the Associated Press. David was bartending at Pinto & Hobbs Tavern, a regular haunt for many of the political staffers, lobbyists, and government workers. I hadn't been living in Albany long, and soon after I walked into the dark bar, I had a creep hitting on me relentlessly.

Once David noticed, he didn't miss a beat. He positioned himself between us, lowered his voice to a slightly menacing level, and said: "Leave my girlfriend alone."

I was stunned, but caught myself, looped my arm through the crook of his elbow, and sat up straight in my chair. "We just started dating," I said, glaring at the creep, who conveniently found a reason to disappear.

David and I grinned at each other and didn't say another word until closing time, at which point he started pouring me free drinks. I helped him clean the bar that first night and we danced to Nina Simone on the jukebox.

He was someone I admired and who I knew would always be in my baby's life.

This felt so right.

I caught David up on the fact that I had been through a few donors, and gave him details on the Conquistador drama, what it was like inseminating in a public restroom with help from The Lawyer, and my obnoxious, red-tape-loving doctor. He listened, rapt. But he was most interested in how it would work for us to get the job done.

I explained how carefully I had been timing my cycles, and that I was on the verge of ovulation. I talked him through the basic procedure: produce sperm, get it all in the menstrual cup without spilling. Hand it off to me, and I'd take it from there.

I was eager to get started, so I gave David the menstrual cup. After he produced the sample and handed it off, I went into one of the bedrooms, inserted the cup, and quickly rubbed one out. David asked about this, inevitably. He had spotted my pink vibrator as I darted into the bedroom to complete my phase of the process.

"I'm not sure how effective it is, but some women on the Facebook groups have this theory that the contractions from orgasming right after insemination can help suck the sperm into the cervix."

"Does that work?!"

"I have no idea. I mean, if women needed to orgasm for the human race to survive, we would be doomed."

David laughed with me. The whole exchange had been weird, yet somehow not awkward. We knew each other so well, were comfortable talking about sex and relationships and everything else in life. I loved how much it didn't feel like a transaction. David wanted nothing but to make my dreams come true.

We made plans for the routine over the next several days. We would do an insemination once per day while I was in Boston. The next one would be the following morning, and the last one just before he drove me to the airport.

David was fascinated by the world of freelance sperm.

"Do you think women wanting to have a baby and get pregnant, but not necessarily going the traditional route . . . do you think that is something that's on the rise? And if so, what's driving it?" he asked.

It was the first time anyone had asked me about why this was happening. I explained that it did appear to be on the rise from what I could see in the Facebook pages. The reason was more complicated. The pandemic certainly played a role, but other factors were also relevant. When it comes to the single mother by choice phenomenon, as much as modern women are focused on their careers and waiting longer to have children, I also think a lot of men in my generation seem much less likely to settle down with one woman—and when they do, they settle down with much younger women.

"Now, if I want to settle down with a guy who's interested in me, half the time he's in his sixties, and he's already had his babies. So, what's my option? At the end of the day, I'm just not willing to wait for men anymore. This is something I want to do."

"And that's amazing," David said. "Honestly, you'd be waiting a while to have kids with someone you just met now, anyway."

It was interesting that David brought this up, as I had done a little bit of dating—almost all first dates only. I had been honest with the guys about my plans to get pregnant, and interestingly, most weren't immediately scared away. I explained to David that several had—comically—suggested that I wait to get to know them, so maybe they could be the father of my baby. Obviously, I told them: "Nope. I'm sorry, but hell no, I'm not waiting for you." I was done waiting for men to be ready to take the next life step with me.

"But if you met someone who you had a genuine connection with and you were both feeling it, maybe that would be a different story?" David asked.

"This would actually be a horrible time to meet somebody that I had a real connection with. Because I don't think desperation in someone's eyes is attractive. And I am legit desperate to have a baby."

David and I spent the next several days eating (he made split pea soup—it was incredible after slow cooking for twenty-four hours) and talking and crying and a little bit of drinking wine. His friend/lover/not-a-boyfriend Kyle came over and the three of us stayed up every night in our pajamas, eating snacks and sharing childhood traumas and funny stories, in equal measure. It felt like home.

In between inseminations, David and I watched movies, danced and sang, and ate his delicious split pea soup until I thought we were going to turn green. Something quieted in my heart. All my anxious focus on getting pregnant was melting away. Now I felt like it would happen. It had to, right?

I CHOSE DAVID BECAUSE I wanted to be able to be certain that I wasn't going to screw up my kid—at least not by using the wrong donor sperm. Life doesn't offer those kinds of guarantees, unfortunately.

Cohen, the bioethicist from Harvard, says there's no easy answers for would-be parents.

He says that it's controversial even just trying to measure whether children of donor conception who are denied a relationship with their biological parent(s) have any resulting psychological deficits.

"You'll see lots of debates in the literature, but the experience of many donor-conceived children I speak to is that they feel something is definitely missing, although that something that is missing is also missing for other children who are the results of sexual encounters with men who are not really part of the picture."

Nationwide, nearly twenty million children—more than one in four—live without a father in the home, according to the US Census Bureau. Less than 6 percent (roughly two million) of American fathers are solo parents, raising their kids on their own. More than 20 percent of American fathers (about seven million) are completely absent from all their children's lives.

The data shows that there can be real consequences for fatherless children when it comes to life outcomes. For example, 71 percent of high school dropouts don't have present fathers; children without fathers are also more likely to struggle academically and score poorly on reading and mathematics; they are also more likely to drop out of school. Kids from fatherless homes are also more likely to engage in delinquency and crime—85 percent of youth in prison have an absent father—and are overall more likely to drink alcohol and abuse drugs in adolescence, have mental health disorders, and have bleaker outcomes in terms of income, unemployment, and homelessness as adults.

This is all very grim, yet Cohen says it shouldn't necessarily influence the decisions people make about who to choose as a co-parent or sperm donor—because that would change which people are conceived and born into the world. That philosophy extends to the debate about whether sperm donors should be allowed to be anonymous.

"This, again, relates to this question of harm," he says. "In a world where we prohibit anonymous sperm donation, the population of men who would become sperm donors is different than in a world where we allow it. As a result, different children come into existence. And so, the idea of benefit and harm is very slippery."

This is the same reason it's difficult for US courts to deal with lawsuits over sperm bank mishaps—cases that are usually settled out of court. If one of the cases ever went to a jury for a verdict, it would be hugely challenging for the families to win, because they would have to argue that there was a "wrongful birth" when their child came into the world. In other words, their child should never have existed. America is a country where individualism is paramount—and stating that someone should never have been born is so contrary to the fundamentals of US culture and jurisprudence, it's unlikely that one would ever be allowed to proceed based on that premise.

In 2017, a family filed a lawsuit, *Norman et al. v. Xytex Corp.*, in Georgia state court, alleging harm because the Xytex Corporation didn't disclose that one of its most popular donors—who has produced at least thirty-six children—had major psychological issues and a criminal background. The child involved in the lawsuit had mental health issues, including suicidal and homicidal thoughts, requiring extensive treatment. The case made it to the Georgia Supreme Court in 2020, which dismissed all claims arising from the child's very existence. However, it did allow one claim to proceed, because it arose from specific impairments to the child that were caused or exacerbated by the sperm bank's alleged wrongdoing. This was a bit of a hollow victory, however, because the recovery available under viable claims against Xytex is likely to be insufficient to finance the plaintiffs' litigation efforts. The Supreme Court of Georgia has, for practical purposes, left the victims of unscrupulous sperm banks "without a remedy," according to a 2022 legal analysis in the *Chicago-Kent Law Review*.

The overall good news for parents of donor-conceived children, courtesy of a study by Golombok that was published in 2023, is that these children are going to be okay: "Contrary to the concerns that have been raised regarding the potentially negative consequences of third-party assisted reproduction for children's psychological well-being, the findings of this longitudinal study point to positive family relationships and child adjustment from childhood to adult life. The findings also suggest that families may benefit from parents of children born through third-party assisted reproduction beginning to speak to their children about the circumstances of their birth at an early age, in an age-appropriate way, ideally before they start school."

Golombok says that the big difference between most fatherless children and those born to single mothers by choice is that, because the latter are planned pregnancies, those mothers tend to have better financial and social circumstances in place to provide support for the child.

The study, published in the journal *Developmental Psychology*, was actually the seventh phase of a longitudinal (multi-year) research effort seeking to determine whether children born through third-party assisted reproduction experienced psychological problems, or difficulties in their relationship with their mothers, in early adulthood.

It also explored the "impact of disclosure of their biological origins, and quality of mother-child relationships from age three onward." The study followed sixty-five assisted reproduction families, including twenty-two surrogacy families, seventeen egg donation families, and twenty-six sperm donation families. These groups were compared with fifty-two unassisted conception families when the children were twenty years old.

The study found little to no differences between assisted reproduction and unassisted conception families in mothers' or young adults' psychological well-being, or the quality of family relationships.

However, researchers did find that mothers who used donor eggs reported less positive family relationships than sperm donation mothers, and young adults conceived by sperm donation reported worse communication between family members than those conceived by egg donation. Young adults of donor conception who were informed about their conception before age seven had less negative relationships with their mothers, and their mothers showed lower levels of anxiety and depression.

The study suggests that sperm donation does not interfere with the development of positive mother-child relationships or psychological outcomes of the child in adulthood.

That's not to say there aren't challenges that arise, or specific considerations that parents of donor-conceived children shouldn't follow. My biggest question was what this all means for the child of a single mother by choice; it doesn't feel good to deny a child a two-parent household.

"Of course, children see around them other families that have either two parents or that have a father, and children who are born to single mothers by choice will start to notice because they don't have either of these things," Golombok says.

"Especially once children go to school, they see other families, and they begin to ask questions," she continues. "Many single mothers by choice have thought long and hard about this issue before pursuing this path."

Golombok was surprised to learn how early children begin to ask questions about why they don't have a father, or why their family is different from other children's families.

"That is an additional challenge for women having children alone," she says. "And it seems to be less of an issue for children with two moms, perhaps because other children see that they've got two parents. Often, we find that children's questioning comes from other children asking them about their family, and sometimes they haven't really seen their families as different until it's pointed out to them."

Golombok also dismissed the notion that people with nontraditional families shouldn't pursue those paths for fear of harming the child or children.

"I don't see why a single person wanting to have children is any more selfish than somebody who's in a relationship with a partner," Golombok says. "The thinking behind it is that children might have problems in some way because of this idea that children need a father to flourish. It reflects a more general view that is still prevalent in our society, that it's important for children to grow up in a traditional family with a mother and father. And if they don't have that, they will be psychologically harmed. It's a common view in our society that some people feel for religious reasons, moral reasons. It was taken for granted that this was the best family setup for children."

Golombok's research at the Centre for Family Research at the University of Cambridge in the United Kingdom has focused on questioning these societal assumptions, which are not always borne out by evidence.

Like with adoption, often the children of donor conception need the information on the donor more than they actually need the relationship, she says. It's part of natural curiosity to wonder if they look like the donor, or have his personality, or whether he likes sports or shares any of their interests.

That's not to say that it can't be beneficial for the children who do have the opportunity to at least meet, or even build a relationship, with their biological father.

"There's huge variation: For some young people, knowing the donor matters an awful lot. It affects how they see themselves; it affects how they develop as a person, who they are," Golombok says. "My view is that donors should be identifiable, because if children or young adults want this information, they should be able to get it. But also bear in mind that, for some, they won't be the slightest bit interested."

My first series of inseminations with David didn't take.

Then, I was incredibly disappointed when I had to cancel the second one because I ovulated right around January 6, 2021, the day of the siege on the US Capitol, which happened a ten-minute walk from my apartment, spilling an angry, MAGA-clad crowd into the streets surrounding me. Between that and the enduring pandemic, I decided to wait until February.

I was so confident that it was meant to be, I couldn't wait to get back to Boston. This time I was staying in a hotel because David's roommate was worried about COVID—understandably; I was traveling on a plane in winter. He came over and did a quick insemination and hung out with me in the hotel room for a bit before he had to leave for work. I stayed in my hotel room and tried to work on my research into the freelance sperm world.

The next day, everything crumbled. David's sperm analysis results had come back. He was infertile.

He texted me, clearly brokenhearted. He apologized, though it wasn't his fault. A screenshot of the results made it clear there was zero hope of getting pregnant with his sperm.

I could tell David was hurting. Even though he had never planned on having a child, it doesn't necessarily feel good to know the option's off the table.

Heartbroken, I cried, alone, in my hotel room. For exactly one hour. Then I gathered myself together and started searching for a new donor back in D.C., on the off-chance that I'd find someone great enough that I could avoid having to miss another cycle. I can't explain the determination that took over my brain and body during this entire fertility journey. Some unseen force has driven me to continue putting one foot in front of the other and my eyes have never wavered from the prize: a baby, a kiddo.

This rushed approach was exactly what I would have advised any other recipient to avoid doing. But faced with the crushing disappointment month after month of tracking my cycle, all for nothing, I knew I wouldn't be able to hold back if I could find someone promising with current STI records who was willing to know the kid from birth.

One donor rose to the top of the pile. His name was Eddie. He was tall, handsome, a bit of a hippie—and he only worked with people who were willing to tell their kids the truth about where they come from; people willing to keep an open door of communication with him. This was significant because Eddie was Mexican American. He understood the importance of connecting the child with their cultural roots. We started rapidly going through my preliminary vetting questions over video chat and agreed to meet in person to discuss whether it made sense to work together. And so, it was with steely determination (and not much else) that I flew back to D.C. to meet my new donor.

Chapter Nine
The Hippie

I MET EDDIE THE DAY after I got back to D.C. He appeared in my doorway, all six feet of him, with curly black hair, heart-shaped pink-tinted prescription glasses, and an enthusiastic grin. He was filthy, covered in dirt because he had been working in the garden all day. He brought me some seeds so we could plant them in my backyard, which was pretty damn adorable—and definitely a clever way into my gardener's heart. I led him down the narrow hallway of my apartment to the main space and gave him a hug before inviting him to sit down in front of a microphone at my blue laminate retro-diner-style kitchen table. Eddie smiled at me across the table, and complimented my art. I had used sheet music to wallpaper one wall of my apartment and had found big antique frames at a garage sale and spray-painted them a glossy black before filling them with gothic art. I poured us each a glass of red wine and we settled in for a talk.

Eddie is Mexican American, which made it more import-ant to me that he be available to my child so that he or she would feel connected to their heritage and have someone in their life to talk about what it means to be Mexican—or even just a brown person in America. Eddie shared my sentiment that this would be important for any child.

He was incredibly patient with me as I recorded the mutual vetting process. The most important thing I wanted to know was his motivation for donating. How could he be sure he wanted to go through with this? His answer was quintessentially Eddie— a bit rambling, utterly sincere, openhearted, and spiritual, thanks to a core sense of connection he feels with others and the universe at large.

Eddie was compelled to become a donor because he always knew he wanted to be a father.

"I definitely want to have some kids that I'm responsible for day in and day out—that's someday, in the future. I never got to meet either one of my grandfathers. And so I always felt like I was missing out on something. I was like, 'Man, I wish I could meet my granddad,' you know. And I always wanted my kids to meet their grandfather."

The urgency to become a father intensified several years ago when his father was diagnosed with leukemia. Eddie started to feel the pressure of finding somebody with whom he could start a family. But this attitude began to put stress on any relationships he was in because his partners (Eddie is polyamorous) weren't ready. The year before he began donating, Eddie was dating someone who became pregnant and ultimately decided not to keep the child. A month later, his father underwent intensive chemo because his leukemia was worsening. He died a few months afterward.

Eddie was devastated.

"It was those two things: I lost a child, and that feeling—
and then literally losing my father—that led me to say, 'Hey,
life is really short. You never know what's going to happen.'
And I want my individual lineage, my soul lineage, to continue, even though I think we're all part of the same soul. I
think it would be really neat to see a version of me go into
the world."

A friend suggested he consider sperm donation, and it was
a new idea for him, but he decided to sit with the concept for
a bit and weigh it seriously.

"Around New Year's that year, something compelled me,"
he said. "I just went on Facebook, and I typed the word 'sperm'
in the search bar to see what would come up."

Eddie discovered dozens of sperm donation groups. After
lurking for a few days, he started putting himself out there as a
donor and commenting on recipient posts offering his services.
Within two months he received more than four dozen requests
to be a donor.

Eddie said he was "definitely not" donating to four dozen
people. He knew he didn't want to be a super-donor, but he
was overwhelmed and touched that so many people considered
him fit to contribute DNA.

"Just seeing that there were so many people out there with
a desire and at a place where they can give a beautiful and
wholesome life to a child was wonderful—and it was really
flattering," he says.

That was the beginning of his path to freelance sperm donation.

"Now the question is, how many kids do I want to help create, how much energy do I want to put forth toward that? I think the number is twelve. I think twelve kids sounds good," Eddie says.

I asked him how he balanced that with such high demand for his swimmers, and how he chose which recipients to help. At first, he didn't know how to say no because he didn't want to hurt recipients' feelings. But he eventually realized ignoring or ghosting people who didn't feel like a good fit was not the kind thing to do.

"There is no particular formula for why a donor picks the recipient," he said. "There are some donors who seem to just donate to whoever. And that's fair and valid for them. For me, even if I don't get to be a part of the child's life, day in and day out, I consider them to be a part of me and my lineage. So I want—when I look at the person, or the people who will be conceiving and raising this human—to be able to get an idea, or a picture, of what this kid's life will be like."

Eddie would ask himself whether he'd be excited to be their kid, whether he thinks the child would grow up happy with the prospective parent(s). He also believes we all have a biologically driven intuition about what kind of person we each would want to mate with, and so he looks for some level of attraction, whether physical, spiritual, or intellectual, to guide him as he chooses recipients.

He's had moments with perfectly lovely couples where things were "weird, energetically," so he decided to move on until he found someone he clicked with. He's also turned down couples who wanted total anonymity and refused to provide any connection between him and the child.

Naturally, I asked him why he chose to donate to me.

"I really like the energy that I received from your eyes and your smile, and I thought that you seemed like a very caring person," Eddie said.

He also liked that my background picture on Facebook was a page from *Be Here Now*, a book about spirituality and freedom by the yogi and spiritual teacher Ram Dass. We shared a deep affection for the book and the messages it contained.

I told you. He's a hippie. But apparently, so am I. It felt like a good fit. And he seemed to agree.

"I also liked the approach that you presented, the scenario of having the biological father known and present. That seems like a really, really exciting avenue," he said.

One of Eddie's firm rules is that he at least wants pictures and video updates of the child. He's not interested in co-parenting but is open to having more of a relationship with the children, if the parents are comfortable with that.

Eddie smiled his movie star grin and leaned back, opening his arms wide and gesturing around at the universe, as he reassured me that we are all interconnected and that he will always want to stay in my child's life. He struck me as a tenderhearted soul, even if a little naïve about the reality of having a kid around. He was also wicked smart, having won a full-ride scholarship to college, where he studied political science. He was working in construction with the goal of eventually building sustainable communities that are environmentally friendly and carbon neutral. He just oozed goodness. I'm not entirely sure he didn't time travel from the set of a Cheech and Chong flick, but I dug the guy's quirky personality and warmth. We had already cleared up major vetting questions, and this meeting was more of a vibe check. The vibe was good. He used my bedroom to produce a sample in a menstrual cup, and I immediately kicked him out so I could insert it.

"If this all goes well, we'll be in touch for a long time," he said. "Hopefully, we're going to develop a really beautiful friendship."

I had a feeling he was right.

EDDIE AND I GREW CLOSE. It wasn't romantic, but a partnership, of sorts. Every cycle he would come over, usually three days in a row, for insemination. It wasn't uncommon for me to make us dinner so we could sit and talk and relax after the insemination. I would make something simple, like meatloaf, or a grilled chicken, tomato, and avocado salad. One night he surprised me by bringing over fixings to prepare pozole, a traditional Mexican stew with hominy, chicken, and fresh avocado. We would drink wine, laugh, and talk about the possibility of me having a baby. What would the baby look like? Would it have his curly hair? My green eyes? I felt like this hippie was just as excited as I was at the prospect of creating a life.

He asked me how I felt when I would meditate after insemination to focus all my energy on encouraging my egg to receive the sperm and let it take root.

"I almost feel like I'm floating," I said. "I feel a warmth in my womb come over me, and I feel connected to the ground, as if my feet have roots in the ground like a tree, but at the same time I'm practically buoyant, and it just feels very, very powerful."

He believed in my ability to manifest this baby and make it real. It was an incredible feeling. I really wanted to believe it was going to work, and that he would be there, in my child's life, from birth.

But gradually, things started shifting. Eddie missed a few inseminations here and there—meaning I would only have one or two fresh sperm inseminations per cycle. Then he missed an entire cycle with me and wasn't very communicative about it until the last minute.

He was getting flaky, and I still wasn't pregnant. I had officially been trying for over a year at this point: one cycle with The Conquistador; six cycles with The Lawyer; two with David; three with Eddie. And it was getting harder to count on Eddie. He was increasingly busy and getting discouraged by our lack of success.

By this point, he had tried with six recipients, including myself, and none of us had gotten pregnant. He was starting to have second thoughts about donating, and I could feel his commitment waning.

It was heartbreaking and frustrating, especially because I was beginning to realize that I would need to move on to IVF soon. At my age you were considered infertile after six months of trying. A year of trying—with most of that being medicated cycles—well, it was worrisome.

My control-freak doctor agreed. It was time. But the problem was he thought I was still working with The Lawyer, the same donor he had tested the sperm of previously.

While Eddie was rethinking his plans to be a sperm donor, I was longing for the stability and predictability of The Lawyer. I started weighing the importance of having a known donor the kid could meet with the basic necessity of a reliable donor who had proven successes. Plus, I was worried it was time to move on to IVF, and Eddie wasn't open to that.

I searched the Facebook groups for other suitable donors in the D.C. area, but so many were inconsistent, or weird, or pressuring me for sex.

Ultimately, I decided to return to The Lawyer, and Eddie and I remained friends. I still question myself about that decision to this day, because it was a moment when I put my desire to become a mother before the best interest of my child. But that child might never exist if I hadn't turned to either The Lawyer or the sperm banks—which felt much more like a crapshoot.

The Lawyer graciously took me back, and was understanding of my reasoning for wanting to work with a donor willing to meet the child. He continued to draw the line on meeting until age eighteen, but agreed to provide much more information than I could have ever gotten through a sperm bank, including family medical history and pictures of him through his childhood and adulthood. We had also forged a friendship of sorts, even staying in touch, occasionally, on political and other newsworthy matters for which we had shared interests.

We agreed to try one more cycle of home insemination before moving on to IVF, but like the other ones, it didn't take. It had been month after month of peeing on sticks to find out when I was ovulating. Day after day of temping, taking medications and dozens of supplements and Chinese herbs that promised to restore my aging eggs. The Lawyer continued to be incredibly kind and patient, but I was fed up.

Chapter Ten
A Hundred Fertility Heartaches

D O YOU HAVE $40,350 TO spare?

That's how much our hypothetical woman—let's call her Rhonda—will need to spend just for a shot at having a baby. Or she could buy a new 2023 Tesla Model 3 in cash. Only one of those two purchases would be a sure thing.

Our Rhonda is a spunky woman with an average job (hot tub sales), above average pay ($65,000, including commission), and a great credit rating (790). She lives in Daytona Beach, Florida, where her cost of living is 3 percent below the national average.

These factors are the only reason Rhonda can even consider embarking on an IVF journey, because she will inevitably be going into some debt along the way.

Rhonda has no fertility coverage, so she'll start by picking a donor and buying her sperm, which comes at an average of $1,000 a pop, plus about $250 for shipping. Most women buy three to five vials of a donor's product at one time because with the shipping charge it's cheaper than paying for one at a time.

It's also just good planning—Rhonda's got a good head on her shoulders. She knows IUI doesn't typically work on the first try, and banks can run out of product from their most popular donors. Rhonda plans to try at least three rounds of IUI before moving on to IVF, so she purchases three vials of sperm for $3,000 plus the $250 for transporting the frozen product. Well, now she's got to pay the clinic's $650 per year storage fee up front for the extra vials she ordered.

Keep in mind that each vial is just one shot at pregnancy—and sperm that's been frozen isn't as healthy as fresh sperm. Plus, one vial of sperm usually contains a fraction of the total donation provided (0.5 to 1 milliliter, compared to the average emission volume of 2 to 4 milliliters, according to Seattle Sperm Bank). Industry officials say that this is because they need to standardize the volume of sperm each client can expect—but it also means they can turn one donation into a bigger profit that has the potential to result in exponentially more babies.

Now Rhonda needs to pay for the procedure, and IUI ranges between $300 to $1,200 each time. Assuming she pays about $600 per IUI, plus about $250 per cycle for the medications that prep her body by first boosting her estrogen and ovulation, and later, her progesterone levels to support implantation of any fertilized egg. Additionally, each time she steps into the doctor's office, she also has to pay $150 out of pocket for the visit. Each cycle would entail roughly five to eight visits, so assuming she goes five times, that's $750. Let's say all three IUIs fail; that means she's spent $7,200 so far, with zero payoff.

That's beyond insurmountable for many Americans—particularly when nearly a third of US adults would struggle to cover a $400 emergency expense. And even people with decent savings accounts would quickly run out of cash for the cost of sperm if they struggled to get pregnant over the course of several months or years.

None of this takes into consideration whether our girl has had to take unpaid leave from work for multiple doctors' visits. Keep in mind, Rhonda counts on making commission on top of her salary. Now she's losing out on sales because she keeps having to show up late or duck out early for her appointments. Plus, she will end up paying interest when she needs to use her credit card and a small loan to cover some up-front costs.

Poor Rhonda has been trying IUI for three straight months at this point. Now thirty-eight, her blood tests show she has low ovarian reserve, meaning she's running out of eggs, and—due to her age—egg quality is also a concern. The doctors recommend moving on to IVF, which is more expensive but has better odds of success.

Let's assume her basic total cost for a full cycle of IVF with all medications comes to $26,400. Don't forget to tack on another $1,250 for a fresh vial of sperm plus shipping. Now, let's say Rhonda was able to get ten eggs from her egg retrieval (the first phase of IVF). That would be a decent number for her age; forty-year-old women produce an average of eight eggs per IVF cycle. The next step is to either put sperm in a petri dish with the egg to let the magic happen, or to have the doctor perform intracytoplasmic sperm injection (ICSI), in which they insert a tiny needle into the egg and inject a single, healthy sperm to increase the odds of success. ICSI costs $800 to $2,500 depending on the clinic and how many eggs you get. Rhonda shells out $2,000, out of pocket, for ICSI on all ten eggs to give herself the best shot at success.

At this point, the doctors and embryologist must wait to see if fertilization is a success. The best-case scenario is for all the eggs to fertilize and then make it to day five in the petri dish—by which point they should be blastocysts (a rapidly dividing cluster of cells ready for transfer into the uterus).

But every step of the way in IVF is a battle against attrition.

Rhonda gets lucky and learns that eight of her eggs fertilized. But then some of them stop growing after a few days, so only six day-five embryos are produced. Then it's time to have the embryos tested genetically, which is not covered by insurance, and typically costs another $350 per embryo, though some clinics will charge a lump sum—say $2,500—for the first four, and $250 each for every subsequent embryo. Rhonda pays $3,000 to have the six blastocysts tested. Of those day-five embryos, Rhonda has three come back normal—and that is a pretty decent outcome.

The basic total cost includes the cost of the embryo transfer, though that, too, can come with extra sticker shock. Most clinics recommend assisted hatching, a process by which they crack the outer "shell" of the embryo to make it more likely that it will implant in the uterus. This averages $500 a pop and is rarely, if ever, covered by insurance. Which brings us to that grand total of $40,350 in out-of-pocket costs for about six months of assisted reproductive treatment.

It's no wonder women turn to the unregulated sperm market.

Keep in mind, Rhonda was juggling mood swings the entire time she was injecting herself with hormones. Her regular life—perhaps going out for drinks with friends, taking rigorous work-out classes, attending networking events, and staying up late to get work done—all goes out the window. She can no longer afford small luxuries (she really couldn't afford them in the first place), and she has to abstain from many joyful aspects of life—drinking, rich food, and late nights—indefinitely, to help increase her chances of success. It's not for the faint of heart.

Along the way, Rhonda survived a hundred little infertility heartaches, dozens of financial panics (including two new credit card applications), and the constant reminder of her body's failures. She may find herself downgrading to a smaller apartment, an older car, or giving up her mani-pedi routine and other splurges to make ends meet. The baby—the one thing she has to look forward to now that she's living like an ascetic—becomes just as high-stakes as it is elusive.

And none of this guarantees a healthy pregnancy resulting in a healthy baby. But let's be nice and assume Rhonda has a first-round IVF success. Rhonda's been through enough. Now she's having twins!

It's hard not to feel like fertility clinics are trying to nickel-and-dime you every chance they get. The first step of any IVF cycle is forking over the money. My own doctor wouldn't even see me or speak by phone to answer a basic question until I had paid for what they said would be my out-of-pocket portion for the entire procedure. I later learned that they overestimated this amount by almost $2,700—which I am certain they knew that they were doing. It also took them two months to pay me back what I was owed after I switched clinics due to my disgust with Dr. Patronizing. Apparently, a few clinics do this. They want the extra cash, so they know they have you locked in and paid for multiple IVF cycles, even if it's well beyond what your insurance company says you owe. It's just one more financial obstacle to parenthood. And it's sleazy as hell.

My HEART SANK AS I ran the numbers. Back in the summer of 2020, when I first set out on this quest, I wanted to be sure I could even afford to have a baby. When people complain about the high cost of the fertility industry, a common retort is that if you can't afford it, then you can't afford children in the first place.

That strikes me as a bogus argument. The median annual income in America was a little over $31,000 in 2019, according to US Census data. That isn't far off from the out-of-pocket cost of one round of IVF. Yet many Americans have successfully raised children on low incomes.

I could already tell that between rent, bills, childcare, food, and basic needs for life, I was going to have a very tight budget as a mom. I also felt resolve. It was going to be tough, but I could do it.

To start, I budgeted at least $2,000 a month for childcare if I stayed in D.C. It was a shocking sum to comprehend. More than my rent. I also could go the route of an au pair. You shell out roughly $9,000 up front—money I could save while pregnant—and then pay just $200 to $250 per week ($800 to $1,000 per month) because you're providing them a place to stay and letting them eat your groceries. However, that would require me to get a bigger place with enough room for the au pair and a nursery. Maybe the cost would shake out about the same?

I also had the option of moving to another, cheaper city. It would break my heart to leave D.C., but you have to make sacrifices as a parent. And a move to Pittsburgh or somewhere else on the smaller side could give me a chance to land a three-bedroom house with a mortgage of $1,200 or less. That would be life-changing.

While I may have been in denial about it at first, paying out of pocket for sperm and fertility care would have been impossible for me to afford after a few unsuccessful rounds of insemination with bank sperm at a fertility clinic. Getting real about my budget with a baby was a necessary and terrifying part of the process.

Low-income people face unique challenges that make them more likely to seek out help in the unregulated sperm donor market. There's the high cost of sperm banks and fertility treatments, but also people on a tight budget often don't have jobs that give them paid time off, meaning they lose money every time they have to go to the doctor's office—and fertility patients are automatically frequent fliers, visiting several times a month for blood work, monitoring, and various procedures and tests. On top of that, they must pay for transportation, and those who already have one or more kid have to arrange and pay for childcare.

If I had been paying for sperm on top of my out-of-pocket costs for fertility medication and medical monitoring, I would have been out roughly $30,000 more than I had actually spent—just on sperm. I never thought it would take so many months for me to get pregnant, but looking back I realized that I would have had to turn to this alternative eventually, regardless of what I wanted.

I still needed to save and pay off some debt before a baby arrived. I make decent money as a journalist, more than I ever expected to earn, actually. But getting pregnant—let alone raising a kid—in a single-income household is no joke.

In the 1942 decision *Skinner v. Oklahoma,* the US Supreme Court declared that procreation is "one of the basic civil rights of man . . . fundamental to the very existence and survival of the race," yet US health insurance plans often don't cover fertility treatments necessary to make building a family possible.

It's estimated that only 24 percent of Americans who need assisted reproductive technology get the help they need. That's because, as Rhonda illustrated, it's incredibly costly.

More than seven million women in the US—about 12 percent of those at reproductive age—experience infertility challenges, according to the CDC. Close to 10 percent of men are infertile or have low fertility.

Assisted Reproductive Technology (ART) is a factor in 2.1 percent of births in the United States, or about half of Europe's rate. European countries tend to have higher proportions of ART births, because more of them view the procedures as essential care and, as a result, publicly fund them. Some of the highest ART birth rates are in Denmark (6 percent), Belgium (4 percent), and Sweden (3.5 percent).

As we've established, assisted reproductive technology is expensive. Yet, historically, most state insurance laws incorporated a definition of infertility that relied on a straight couple having unprotected sex for six to twelve months (depending on the woman's age) before coverage kicks in. This automatically excludes gay couples and single people from mandated fertility coverage, meaning they're automatically going to pay more for access to the same reproductive opportunities. New Jersey tried to take on the issue in 2018 by amending its law to provide coverage for single or lesbian women that takes effect once they go through several unsuccessful IUIs. However, while that change gives gay couples a path to pregnancy via ART, it still means they automatically end up paying more than a straight couple.

Beyond that, many gay and lesbian couples say they don't always feel their needs are met or prioritized in traditional fertility clinics designed around the needs of heterosexual couples. And some report experiencing poor treatment from physicians who seem to harbor bias against same-sex couples who express a desire to have a child. For some, this is enough to drive them straight into the open arms of the unregulated sperm market.

A Hundred Fertility Heartaches

. . .

MONIQUE HAD NO IDEA THAT coming out to her lifelong gynecologist would create an obstacle on her road to becoming a mother. But the moment that the doctor met Monique's wife, the woman retreated into vague, evasive half-conversations and refused to answer questions or provide any guidance on finding a sperm donor. After several fruitless visits during which she attempted to extract some guidance on sperm banks, fertility testing, and prenatal vitamins, Monique realized: It was homophobia.

She switched doctors, and eventually gave up relying on the medical industry altogether. Instead, she found her way to the world of freelance sperm. With the help of longtime donor Ron, Monique and her wife now have a nine-month-old daughter. It was an unorthodox step, but one that paid off.

"Now that I've got my daughter, everything that I've ever done makes sense," she says.

LGBTQ+ couples face what bioethicists call "social infertility"—meaning they aren't necessarily biologically unable to reproduce, but their sexual preferences make it impossible to have a baby with their chosen partner.

This thrusts lesbians who want kids into the assisted reproductive industry—or the alternative sperm world—before they even get a chance to find out if they have what it takes to get pregnant naturally.

Some recipients feel freelance sperm donation can fulfill the needs of LGBTQ+ populations more effectively, and without the same experience of prejudice and paternalistic attitudes found in some traditional medical settings.

A unique grief can occur with some lesbian partners because they cannot—at least where science is currently—have a baby that shares both of their DNA. A lesbian couple will never just "accidentally" get pregnant or be able to take the advice to "stop trying so hard" and "let things happen." They will never have a surprise bun in the oven. Every step of the way must be paved with intention and grueling effort.

That was the case for Kelly, who went through three rounds of IVF with no success before meeting her now-wife, Bett. The doctors eventually diagnosed Kelly with adenomyosis, a condition in which endometrial tissue in the lining of the uterus starts growing into the wall of the uterus. It enlarges the uterus, can cause heavy menstrual bleeding, and makes it harder to get pregnant. Ultimately, Kelly had to have a hysterectomy to treat the condition.

She was still hoping to have a biological child by having Bett carry a baby made from Kelly's eggs (she still had her ovaries). Ultimately the couple opted against this, because Bett was concerned about going through such a complex medical procedure.

They wound up finding a freelance sperm donor who got Bett pregnant via AI during their first cycle of home insemination. After having a son, the couple now has a second baby on the way with help from the same donor.

It hasn't all been easy, though. Kelly struggled with serious depression after the baby was born. She yearned to breastfeed and forge a birth-mother-like bond with her son. But her pain was at times invisible to the medical professionals around the couple, because they were focused only on the physical and emotional health of Bett as the gestational mother.

"I had a deep sadness," Kelly said. "I experienced postpartum depression for a few months after he was born. Not being the one to carry and my wife breastfeeding made it emotionally harder because the baby wants the person their milk is coming from all the time."

Eventually Kelly worked through her feelings, and over time has forged a deeper bond with her son. However, it would have been nice if her needs had been addressed during the many follow-up appointments after the baby was born. Medical professionals should be trained to pay closer attention to the mental health needs of the non-gestational or nonbiological parent in same-sex relationships.

Now the couple's son is eight months old, and each day the bond Kelly has with him continues to grow. His regular diet of breast milk is being supplemented with formula, which means that Kelly can take him out on her own without being dependent on her wife for breastfeeding.

"I feel much closer to him as his mom now," Kelly says.

"SURELY THERE MUST BE A waiver?" I was not very successful at concealing my outrage, but I didn't want to take it out on the nurse standing in front of me. The nurse at my fertility clinic glanced behind me at the growing line of people. I didn't care.

I wasn't walking away until I fully understood what she was saying.

"No. I'm afraid not. Dr. Patronizing never lets the single women skip the psych evaluation," she said firmly, clearly not thrown by my barely contained fury.

I scowled at the large sign behind the nurse's head, which bore the clinic's slogan: "Making families, one couple at a time." It was one more reminder that they weren't interested in serving people like me. Every single time I came to the clinic they would ask me where my husband was. I felt I didn't belong there.

Single women are perhaps the biggest population found in this world of unregulated sperm donation. I have no doubt that experiences like those I had at my first clinic play a role in many women choosing this route. At least going with a freelance sperm donor allows us to take our fertility into our own hands.

Single women are frequently subjected to psychological tests before being allowed to obtain fertility treatment, and we routinely encounter judgment for pursuing motherhood alone. Couples aren't expected to jump through the same hoops. After a while it starts to feel like punishment, a conspiracy to teach us all a lesson for not marrying young when our eggs were plentiful and fresh.

Before reaching a decision to go it alone, many single women go through a lengthy process of grieving the future and the family they thought they would have had. Giving up on having a baby with a partner is incredibly difficult for many women, me included. And once they make the leap, they are then reminded that they are "other" every step of the way.

A Hundred Fertility Heartaches

I realized, thanks to Dr. Patronizing, that a woman could be married to a man who beats her, starves her children, and kicks puppies, yet no psychological screening is necessary before she's allowed to shell out many thousands of dollars for the privilege of reproduction.

The psychiatrist who vetted me told me he thought the requirement was idiotic, too. He was personally offended on my behalf that I had to go through such an invasive, condescending, and paternalistic process just to become a mother.

We spoke for about a half hour about my thought process in becoming a mother. He asked whether I had considered the child's perspective about being donor-conceived; how I would handle questions from the child about their origin; what my thinking was in choosing my donor; and what I wanted in terms of a relationship from my known donor. At the end he said he would be happy to write me a letter saying I was fit for parenthood. He even sent it to me in advance and gave me a chance to review and edit it before he submitted it to my doctor—that's how disgusted he was with the gatekeepers of the system.

Essentially two men—my fertility doctor and a psychologist—exchanged notes and agreed between the two of them that the former could accept outrageous sums of money to attempt to get me pregnant. I was not a part of that discussion. This felt so gross and so wrong, I don't know where to begin to explain the yuck factor. But I had checked the box, passed go, and was on my way to getting some fertility help.

Of course, I had to pay this psychologist for his assessment—just one more unfair cost to single women when you go the traditional clinical route.

JENNIFER IS "ONE OF THOSE freaks" who always wound up at the children's table at any social gathering, talking and playing with the kids.

"I just love kids," says the brunette with big brown eyes. "I love other people's kids. I fall in love with them too easily. I always knew that I was going to have kids in my life. I've never particularly dreamed of having a partner, but I dreamed of kids."

Jennifer veers between the vibe of a gentle schoolteacher and that of a fiery, authoritative voice on donor-conceived rights, depending on her mood.

The oldest of three children from a Christian family in the Deep South, Jennifer knew by junior year of high school that if she didn't meet a man to settle down with, she would eagerly become a single mom. At the time she only had a vague idea of what that meant or how it would work—assuming it must involve a sperm bank and some high-tech medical intervention.

Solo motherhood was essentially "Plan A." As Jennifer points out, it can be pretty nice not having to negotiate things like discipline, private versus public schools, or diet. The thirty-eight-year-old is now a solo mom by choice of two who loves her life just the way it is.

Jennifer got her fertility checked in her mid-thirties, and when her numbers came in on the lower side, the doctor called her and said, "Ma'am, if you want to have a kid you and your husband need to start trying now."

"I was like, 'Well, clearly you didn't read my file,'" Jennifer says, laughing. Over the next year she worked on getting her business to a place where she could work as a consultant so she could live wherever she wanted and started paying for her own health insurance.

Then she was ready.

When her pregnancy dreams didn't work out after a few rounds of home insemination with her gay best friend from college, she turned to the world of unregulated sperm donation— not because it was her only option as a single person with one income, but because it was her preference after researching the experiences of donor-conceived people.

"It was important to me to know about the person who my kid's other half would be coming from," she says. "Because I do think that that matters. I think that matters a lot."

She also liked being able to personally vet the donors, whether she found them online or through friends of friends. And she was clear on what she wanted.

"I started thinking: 'Who in my life has characteristics I would want for a genetic father of my children?' Someone creative, someone ambitious, someone curious," Jennifer says.

"I was lucky in that a lot of people said yes and were willing to try to help me. I was unlucky in that a lot of people don't understand how fertility works and the logistics were horrible," she adds. "No one can ever be available when you need them."

Jennifer also perused the Facebook groups and Just a Baby, even Coparents.com—a site where people find each other to conceive and raise a baby together in a non-romantic partnership.

"I had the most success just putting up a dating profile: 'Single white woman seeking sperm donor with [these characteristics]. If you're interested and want to know more, reach out,'" she said.

Jennifer got pregnant for the first time with the help of a known donor who she found through her post on a dating app.

However, when she went in for her noninvasive prenatal testing (NIPT), she learned the baby had a genetic anomaly that would lead to severe disability and likely early death. She made the incredibly difficult decision to terminate for medical reasons.

"People don't talk about termination for medical reasons, at all," she says. "I think about my son all the time. I think about this little person who was in my body that I never got a chance to meet, and I was in a very lonely place for a while because it's not something people want to talk about."

Eventually Jennifer switched to a sperm bank donor after a lengthy stint in the realm of freelance sperm. She said the whole idea of a bank weirded her out—far more than accepting sperm from strangers. It also made her realize how sperm banks encouraged her to look at completely different criteria from what she really cared about. She still prioritized personality more than appearance, but the banks weren't set up to clearly provide that kind of information.

"There aren't checkboxes for curiosity and ambition and creativity. How do you find that in someone at a sperm bank?" she says.

She ended up finding a donor who she liked because he was a bit older and seemed like he might grasp the gravity of creating life through sperm donation. She bought five vials of his OpenID-at-eighteen sperm and started trying to get pregnant with home insemination—she had no desire to go through a clinic. She got pregnant on the third home insemination cycle, and her daughter was born via C-section in March 2020, "ten days before the world shut down."

"They put her little head next to mine, and it was just like everything made sense and felt at peace and at ease in the world. I did it," Jennifer says. "Something I've been working toward for so long had finally, finally happened."

Even before her daughter was born, Jennifer had started tracking down other parents who had conceived half-siblings with the same sperm donor via Facebook groups and the Donor Sibling Registry. Quickly she realized there were at least thirty families out there with kids who were half-siblings to her daughter. It was something she had hoped to avoid by using a freelance sperm donor who had some self-imposed limits.

"It was a lot," Jennifer says. "I am one of the admins for our Facebook group for our donor family. I'm sort of the self-appointed family historian and keeper of all the numbers and facts because someone has to do it until the kids are old enough to own it for themselves. None of us really know how many kids there are out there from our donor."

She does like being able to connect with the parents of her daughter's siblings and feels part of a bigger, extended family. Roughly half of the families are queer, most of the rest are solo moms by choice, plus there are two heterosexual families. The Facebook family group took off at the beginning of COVID and all the families' kids were young, so the families formed bonds around the trauma of being stuck at home with little ones. There have been challenges, however.

"There have been some really awkward political issues. There are some pro-Trump people who are now family. I would not be friends with them in real life, but they are family now because their children are related to my children and we stay connected because of that," she says.

Jennifer was surprised to discover how profoundly she felt the new connections.

"I did not expect to care so deeply. But when I'm looking at these donor siblings, I see my kids in them. And it feels like family. It feels very naturally like family."

By the time her first child was nine months old, Jennifer decided to try for a second baby. She knew she wanted it to be the same donor, and that IVF was off the table, financially. It took her two cycles of home insemination before she became pregnant with her second daughter, who was born in November 2021.

Recently she's been trying for a third and final child.

Jennifer has one more vial left of her donor's sperm and is planning to attempt a home insemination with the help of a midwife when her travel schedule settles down.

"Something was missing from my life, and it wasn't a partner. It was another kid," she says.

Jennifer's certainty and single-minded pursuit of her dreams inspired and reassured me. Even though she ultimately went with a sperm bank donor, Jennifer chose the solo mom life and is making it work every day.

Her story reminded me that everyone who ventures into the unregulated sperm market—or single motherhood—is there because they have no other choice.

Chapter Eleven
Congratulations, You're a Father

Trent Arsenault couldn't have expected federal agents to appear at his door, demanding to search his home.

But in 2010, the self-described Christian virgin became the first-ever private sperm donor to be targeted for FDA enforcement.

The FDA's Center for Biologics Evaluation and Research (CBER) sent Arsenault a cease-and-desist order and threatened him with a $100,000 fine due to his prolific private donations. That same year, agents appeared at his door and searched his home on four separate occasions. The California man made 328 donations to forty-six different recipients with the intent to get them pregnant. At the time, his efforts had resulted in fourteen births (the number later rose to at least twenty-five, as Trent continued donating throughout the federal enforcement action). Although he abstained from sex, Trent had STI testing every six months and had been providing fresh sperm, primarily to lesbian couples, free of charge since 2006.

CBER said that because Trent failed to provide his donations through a bank or clinic and hadn't had the extensive (and expensive) weekly testing and the mandatory six-month freeze and quarantine of sperm that all sperm donors must complete, he was in violation of federal laws and regulations governing donation of biological tissue.

Yet despite wide evidence of even more prolific donors in operation today, the FDA has not gone after a single freelance sperm donor since Trent was forced to shut down his personal operation more than a decade ago.

Now that freelance sperm donation is exploding, the agency will soon need to grapple with how—and if—it plans to regulate this growing form of reproductive activity among private Americans. CBER's sole foray into the fray via Trent's case only served to raise an uncomfortable ethical and legal question for the agency, which may be the reason no freelance sperm donor has been targeted in the same way since: "Under what circumstances can the government tell you not to conceive with another person?"

The FDA's strict and costly regulations around donating sperm with a known donor aren't required when the man is a "sexually intimate partner" of the recipient. The problem is that the federal government has no clear definition for a sexually intimate partner—an omission that became central in the proceedings in Trent's case. In fact, CBER asserted in that case, "The plain meaning of the words . . . do not require further explanation."

Trent and others contend that having had someone's sperm in your body via artificial insemination qualifies them as a sexually intimate partner, and that continued exposure to that person's sperm for the purposes of getting pregnant would pose no additional risk to the recipient, nor would it violate laws governing tissue donation.

This argument is key for Trent and all freelance sperm donors, but also because recipients who want to work with a known sperm donor but go through a clinic—say, instead of the backseat of a Volkswagen—could also forgo the costly testing, freezing, and six-month quarantine that would otherwise be required prior to IUI or IVF. This also could help eliminate requirements at some clinics for psychological evaluations and copies of the legal contract, among other bureaucratic indignities.

Trent's interpretation is actually the law of the land in his home state of California, meaning in that state, one home insemination achieves sexually intimate partner status for any given donor-recipient pair.

Unfortunately, the FDA held that Trent's assertions about how to define "sexually intimate partner" were merely an effort to skirt the issue, and in 2012 he was ultimately barred from donating, unless and until he complied with FDA requirements and obtained written permission from the agency.

In the absence of federal clarity, many US fertility clinics conflate the idea of sexually intimate partners with romantic partners who will act as a parent to the child. They therefore don't allow the use of fresh sperm from private sperm donors, who otherwise would fit the California criteria for a sexually intimate partner, for fear of FDA enforcement and getting ensnared in later legal battles between donor and recipients over child support and custody. Some clinics even require sexually intimate partners to sign a contract saying both people will parent the child. This interpretation—which I would argue is erroneous—creates major obstacles for women who want to make their own choices about who to use as a sperm donor and establishes a clear risk that many gray-market donors may not have considered.

Some have called for regulation or tougher enforcement to somehow limit super sperm donors like Trent. That's unlikely to happen for a pretty good reason, says Judith Daar, the former chair of the ethics committee for the American Society for Reproductive Medicine, a professional group representing medical providers in the fertility industry.

"Americans don't have an appetite for regulating natural reproduction," Judith says, though abortion appears to be the exception. "We, as a society, do feel like we need to honor people's decisions about how many children they want to have and with whom they have them. It's not that I think that it's terrific for a donor to be responsible for dozens or hundreds of offspring. I'm just saying, as long as we're going to make rules about what donors can do in the reproductive arena, we should be considering everyone and treating them equally."

Admitting someone is a sexually intimate partner in one state could actually help support the legal argument in another state that the donor is a father to the donor-conceived child. Each of the US's fifty states has a different set of governing donor conception. Meaning, what worked for your friend in Oregon may not apply in Vermont or Florida or Texas. Recipients need to do research into their home state to learn what their local laws dictate.

"One of the most ridiculous legal decisions I've ever read came out of Virginia's Court of Appeals, in a case where a single mother by choice did a home insemination with a guy friend," says Deborah Wald, a San Francisco–based family law specialist. "She used a turkey baster, and under Virginia law, they define assisted reproduction as an insemination using a medical implement. The court found that a turkey baster is not a medical implement; it's a kitchen implement, and therefore he was the legal father."

The April 2015 court decision stemmed from a verbal deal that Joyce Rosemary Bruce struck with Robert Preston Boardwine. Robert provided free sperm and Joyce used the turkey baster, eventually becoming pregnant in 2010. Her theory was that avoiding sex would protect her parental rights and designate Robert as a donor. Robert's theory was that he would have an active role and be involved in making major decisions about raising the child. They did not have a contract outlining their intentions.

"There really is no shortcut to doing this the right way," adds Deborah, who wrote the California law governing known sperm donors and defining sexually intimate partners.

The former friends had a falling-out after Joyce declined to use Robert's suggestion as a name for the child. They didn't see each other for five months, until Robert visited Joyce in the hospital after the boy was born.

Afterward, Joyce said visits with Robert were uncomfortable, and when she tried to end all contact, he went to court, where Joyce's case fell apart—all due to the instrument of insemination.

"The path to fatherhood may have been unconventional," the court said, but Robert's parental rights must be preserved.

Stories like these worried me, so I initially tried to find a way to use a freelance sperm donor in a fertility clinic, but many don't accept the more liberal definition of a sexually intimate partner. As a result, recipients must jump through major hoops.

That includes thousands of dollars of testing and a six-month quarantine of the sperm, meaning the sperm must be tested prior to freezing, then remain frozen for six months before it (and the donor) are retested for infectious disease (all at the cost of the recipient). Obviously, this significantly delays fertility treatment—which matters when you're of "advanced maternal age," which is anything over thirty-five.

Unfortunately, the US Food and Drug Administration hasn't caught up with California, and there's no indication the agency will sharpen its definition of sexually intimate partners anytime soon.

EARLY ON IN MY OWN journey, I contacted Meryl Rosenberg, a Maryland-based attorney who specializes in assisted reproductive law and who helped write that state's legislation on those issues. She drafted my contract with The Conquistador.

Our first conversation had my head spinning. Meryl would have preferred I go through the official "directed donor" FDA process, red tape and all, but she wasn't fazed or judgmental when I told her I would be doing home insemination with a donor I found on an app.

"That's fine, as long as it's artificial insemination," she said. "It is AI, isn't it?" Technically, this last sentence was a question, but it had the stern tone of a demand.

I, of course, agreed, because at that stage, that's what The Conquistador and I had planned for.

From there, Meryl ran through a multiverse of potential futures for myself and my child, and then she quizzed me on how to handle any number of these (generally terrible) circumstances.

"What if you die?"

"Not sure yet. I'm still deciding who the kiddo would live with."

"No, I mean, if you die, would the donor be interested in becoming a parent at that point? Would you want that?"

Yikes. I had no idea how I felt about that.

"Uh . . . pass! I need to talk to him about that."

"Will the person you designate to take custody of any resulting children be willing to honor your wishes to allow ongoing contact with the donor? Will you choose someone who lives close to him to make that possible?"

Damn, Meryl, get off my jock, I thought, equal parts amused and terrified by the galaxy of new things to worry about that had just started unfolding in my mind.

"I definitely want whoever I choose to maintain contact between the child and the donor. But I can't dictate where they live until my kid is eighteen. I mean, I'll be dead."

"What if your donor helps you produce a child, but later learns he can't have any more biological children, for whatever reason? Would he consider pursuing custody if that was the case?"

"I'm going to start writing these down," I said.

These are the kinds of pitfalls that having a lawyer can help you avoid. I wouldn't have had these conversations with any of my donors without Meryl's guidance.

"I don't think there's a one-size-fits-all contract," she said. "I do think there are plenty of known donation arrangements out there that work; so long as the donor knows they're a donor, not a parent, then there's no reason that can't be worked out. But you want to make sure that everybody is on the same page."

Meryl emphatically encourages prospective parents to go to a lawyer to have their contracts drafted—she says it takes a professional to accurately sort out exactly what does and doesn't need to be included.

To protect everyone's interests equally, the donor and recipient must each have separate lawyers—typically both are paid for by the recipient, though The Conquistador generously paid for his own, as some donors do.

Meryl said there were risks to maintaining a relationship between the donor and the child, though she noted that there's a tension between what's right according to the law and what's right for the child, or in the context of psychology and child development. Regardless of the level of contact agreed upon, both parties are linked for life, and precautions must be taken.

"Don't leave room for the child to call the donor 'Dad,'" Meryl says. "It's a slippery slope. I caution people—the more that the donor behaves as a parent, the more ammunition they have to try to challenge custody."

With all the genetic testing and screening that's available out there, if the kid eventually wants to find answers, there's not going to be much you can do to prevent that, she says.

It's critical that everyone is clear that the intended parent is the ultimate decider on all child-related matters, even if there's an ongoing relationship. That's how you avoid a situation like that of Joyce and Robert, who will now be co-parenting their child for the rest of their lives.

Any deviation from the agreed-upon parameters can have disastrous effects on a person's livelihood and family relationships.

ARI NAGLE IS A WELL-TRAVELED super-donor whose life looks fairly glamorous. It's not uncommon for him to post pictures of himself—sometimes sipping champagne—from what appears to be first class as he's headed to produce more offspring or visit his donor children in some new, exotic destination.

The unglamourous reality: His wages are being garnished to help pay for the needs of nine different children from five different mothers. Four of those were cases where a single mother fell on hard times and the state went after him to offset the welfare expenses for the child. More than half of Ari's salary goes to child support. He struggles financially and it impedes his ability to donate to other women who need his help.

Ari might not have this problem if the FDA defined sexually intimate partners as two people who have exchanged bodily fluids. Such a change would ease the restrictions on allowing known donors to work with recipients through clinics and could potentially make it easier to be legally considered a sperm donor through home insemination—as long as pregnancy attempts were done via AI.

Despite his financial troubles, Ari says he's not bitter about the women who came after him for child support.

"It doesn't surprise me that some women went back on their word. What's more surprising is that out of seventy moms, only five of them sued. That's shocking," he says.

Ari recently had a mother of a one-year-old baby ask him for $50 to help with a $250 hospital bill. While he would have liked to pay the whole thing, he couldn't even spare that small portion.

Ari's experience has been a serious cautionary tale among more up-and-coming donors, who are increasingly skeptical about signing contracts. Many say it's just handing over blatant evidence of paternity that will only serve to get them in front of a family court judge in record time.

FROM THE BEGINNING, THE LAWYER and I had a legal contract in place to make sure that we were both protected. But, as far as the clinic was concerned, he was my boyfriend.

The Lawyer was very concerned about me coming after him for child support, and I wanted to make sure he would never challenge me for custody. Having to say on paper that he was my boyfriend put us both in a vulnerable position—but we trusted each other. It wasn't something either of us took lightly.

Whether or not to use a contract is one of the most hotly debated topics on the Facebook pages. One camp believes a contract can be a valuable tool to help the recipient and donor establish what the intent of all parties was at the time of insemination. The anti-contract faction argues that signing a document that explicitly outlines who is the biological father of a child is more of a legal liability than a legal help. I've spoken to several donors who wound up paying child support after a recipient used a contract as evidence that they were the biological father of the children in question.

Many recipients pull contracts off the internet instead of paying a lawyer (I paid $1,000 for mine). But this can be risky because of the vastly different laws governing known sperm donation from one state to the next—an important consideration if you ever anticipate moving with your child. Plus—and I know this will blow your mind—you're not a lawyer. You do not know how to protect yourself and your child the way a professional can. As someone who resents spending money just to get pregnant, I say: Shell out the money. When has something ever mattered more?

Deborah Wald, the San Francisco–based family law specialist who wrote the law in California that governs using known sperm donors, has been watching the growing trend of unregulated online sperm donation with concern and skepticism.

"As an attorney, I find freelance sperm donation very scary," Deborah says. "Partly because it really does create an opportunity for people to skip doing their due diligence. And partly because people just pull contracts off the internet, or they don't even bother with any contract at all."

Thanks, in part, to Deborah, it's possible to get a secure contract in California for home insemination with a known donor—even as a single mother. That's relevant because in most of the US, family courts will generally err on the side of giving a child two parents when the donation doesn't go through a bank. Even if one of those biologic parents was intended only to be a sperm donor. This can result in custody challenges and child support payments—and trauma for a child whose life has been upended by poor planning and a legal system that has yet to catch up with the nature of their conception.

For decades, Deborah has been on the front lines, trying to expand the rights and protections for folks in the LGBTQ+ community who want to become parents through gamete donation. She has also represented and drafted contracts for many single mothers by choice and known sperm donors.

Deborah is one of the attorneys who has the dubious responsibility of getting to clean up the messes made when people don't follow the law and use legitimate contracts.

"Lawyers come in two varieties—pilots or janitors," she says. "The job of a pilot is to get you safely to your destination.

And the job of a janitor is to clean up the mess. There's more money in being a janitor, but almost all of us who do assisted-reproduction law would much prefer to be pilots. The whole internet sperm situation is skipping the pilots, instead creating a lot of work for janitors."

Deborah doesn't hide her exasperation or mince words when she sees corners cut by recipients and donors. And she's seen everything.

Once, she received a call from a serial sperm donor who was in disbelief because one of his recipients came after him for child support.

"You guys didn't do your due diligence, you had sex," she recalls telling the man. "You're not a sperm donor, you're a father, congratulations."

By the time this donor reached out to Deborah for help, it turned out he had fathered ten kids.

"It's scary that people think that uttering the words 'sperm donor'—or writing them on a makeshift contract—is enough to make it legally true. But there's really no state in the country where that is true," she says.

Deborah is highly aware of the debate between AI and NI, and she's not amused.

"There is no state in the country where having sex to make a baby qualifies as assisted reproduction," Deborah says. "If you have sex with a guy to make a baby, he is the father of your child."

That means your child is even more vulnerable to custody fights if the donor later wants to be a part of the kids' life.

One piece of advice that I wasn't thrilled to hear: Allowing your donor to have a relationship with your child can actually make you vulnerable to custody challenges—even if you have a contract and conceived through artificial insemination at home or with a doctor's help.

The law should protect these new types of families. Donors should be able to interact with their offspring without fear of paying child support. And recipient parents should be able to give their children access to a relationship with their biological father without having to put their entire family structure in jeopardy. The fact is, the law often does not keep up with the realities of human behavior.

"People are winging it. And sometimes it works," Deborah says. "I have friends who did fairly casual sperm donation and it worked great. But we have a system in many states at this point where there is a way to do it right. And if you do it right, then the words in the contract are actually legally enforceable. And my concern with the freelance version is people aren't taking the time to understand what it would take to do it right in their specific state."

Doing it "wrong" can have devastating consequences.

KRIS WILLIAMS TEARS UP EASILY when speaking about the nearly four-year-old son she hasn't seen in almost two years, since losing a custody battle with her ex-wife and having her status as the child's mother stripped from his birth certificate.

"I watch the old home videos and cry," says the self-described fifty-one-year-old butch lesbian. "I miss him very much and I worry about what he went through when she took me away from him."

Kris wonders if he remembers her.

When the Supreme Court made gay marriage the law of the land in the landmark 2015 case, *Obergefell v. Hodges,* parental rights were part of the package.

Those rights where bolstered the same year in *Pavan v. Smith,* when the Supreme Court ruled that states must extend the same rights that heterosexual couples have to queer couples when it comes to listing the non-gestational parent on the birth certificate. The legal opinion is that queer parents are entitled to the same presumption of parenthood given to straight married couples. This was a major victory for LGBTQ+ couples.

Yet gay couples remain uniquely vulnerable in lower-level courts across the country.

Kris is currently living the worst-case scenario for a non-gestational lesbian mother in America.

In February 2023, the Oklahoma County District Court found that Kris did not have legal rights to the child that her ex-wife, Rebekah Wilson, had conceived with donor sperm.

"The implications are harsh because this case is devastating. It's ripping a family apart," said Rob Hopkins, the Oklahoma attorney representing Kris.

The court found that because Kris had never legally adopted the child, she was not legally a parent and had no rights under Oklahoma law. The judge said that she hadn't taken the necessary step to cement her legal relationship to the child.

"My body instantly started shaking," Kris told *The 19th,* a not-for-profit news website. "I mean, pure terror, as a queer person, to be erased."

The women were together for a few years when they found Harlan Vaughn, an online sperm donor, to help them conceive a child. Rebekah conceived the couple's son, and the women were married a few months before he was born. Both their names were put on the birth certificate.

Two years later, Rebekah filed for divorce, moved in with Harlan, and sued to have Kris's name struck from the birth certificate. She also sought to have Harlan named the legal father of the child.

Kris was blindsided, saying Harlan had always presented himself as a gay man (though he later stated in court that the relationship with Rebekah was romantic).

Rebekah and Harlan have since had a second child.

When asked why she didn't attempt to adopt the child, Kris says, "Why should I?"

Judges are finding that birth certificates don't have the full force and weight of the law behind them, says Colorado attorney Ellen Trachman, who specializes in assisted reproduction law and hosts a podcast called *I Want to Put a Baby in You!*

Other states don't necessarily have to rely on just the birth certificate, she adds. However, there are remedies for that: Lawmakers in Colorado passed a law in 2022 that streamlines the adoption process for parents of donor-conceived children to make it faster and easier, with fewer hoops to jump through.

The LGBTQ+ community is concerned that the Oklahoma court decision could create a dangerous precedent that might put other queer parents at risk of losing their children. The case is expected to be appealed. Kris's attorney says that non-gestational parents should always adopt—though he resents this need for an additional step that is not required for heterosexual couples.

For now, Kris says she can't allow herself to imagine the day she is reunited with her son.

"That's just going to get me stuck, not that it hasn't crossed my mind," she says. "When I know that day is coming, I'll start to prepare. Until then, I can't just sit in a sorrow that doesn't allow me to move."

Chapter Twelve

Coming Out of the Conception Closet

WHY, EXACTLY, ARE YOU CHOOSING this particular medication protocol for my IVF cycle?" I asked Dr. Patronizing.

I was back in his sterile office after shelling out more than $6,000—with insurance—before he would even answer any of my questions.

"Because I have thirty-four years of experience getting women pregnant," Dr. Patronizing said, predictably. He was gazing at me from across his desk as I studied the multitude of degrees and certificates hanging on the seafoam-green walls of his office.

"That doesn't really answer my question," I said. "What are your thirty-four years of experience telling you about why I should use this protocol?"

"It's because of your age!" he said, rolling his eyes before he patted his desk and abruptly stood, signaling that our four-minute appointment was over. I remained seated and raised my eyebrow, sternly. He sighed and sat back down. I still had questions.

Dr. Patronizing had just explained that he was going to max me out by using the highest possible recommended doses of three different fertility medications that cost many thousands of dollars (though, thanks to my insurance, I paid about $170 per cycle). I only wanted him to walk me through a semi-scientific explanation behind pumping that level of hormones into my body. The same man who required me to take an invasive psych exam couldn't be bothered to talk me through the reasoning behind his professional opinion. Despite standing my ground and asking him a few more questions, I left the clinic that day with my head spinning.

FOR ME, THE PROCESS STARTED when I went through a specialty mail-order pharmacy to get my fertility drugs. They arrived—signature required—in a massive box loaded with ice packs and more syringes and alcohol pads than any one person should ever need in their lifetime. I gleefully unpacked the pricey drugs, which were: Gonal-F, a follicle-stimulating hormone that spurs the ovaries to grow more than one egg at once; Menopur, a dual-hormone treatment designed to stimulate egg growth; and Letrozole, a hormone used in some chemotherapy treatments that is also used to stimulate egg development. This is not necessarily what every woman going through IVF will be prescribed. Doctors tailor treatments to individuals based on their needs and medical history.

On day one of starting my period I had to call the clinic to notify them I was bleeding and then come in first thing the next morning. They used a vaginal ultrasound (joy) to look at my ovaries and see how many eggs I was cooking.

They sent me home and called me that afternoon to tell me to start injections.

I sat down at my kitchen table in April 2021 for my first injections. It was an incredibly complex process and terrifying to stick needles into myself. But I quickly got the hang of it. For the Menopur, I had to combine five different vials together with sterile water, mix it all up, and then suck it into a syringe that I injected into my lower abdomen. The Gonal-F looked like a pen that also gets injected in my lower abdomen, though I switched up the sides to avoid getting too sore. The Gonal-F came in a red-and-white package and had a handy system where you turned a crank on the back of the "pen" until it reaches the doctor-prescribed dose (three hundred international units for me). Then you simply inject yourself by depressing the plunger. I took the Letrozole in pill form once a day.

At first, I didn't notice anything. Maybe a little bloating. But I soon found myself getting extremely emotional. Word of advice: Keep an eye on yourself during this time. I got a little worked up when the publication that employed me ran an op-ed by a woman who had an insulting and condescending attitude toward professional women who have children, stay-at-home moms, and those who choose not to have children. Forget the idea of being an American career woman who can "have it all"—the message in this essay was: No matter what life choices you make, you're probably a failure.

I was hopped up and riding high on the hormone super-highway when I wrote a lengthy and indignant letter to my then-editor-in-chief, questioning not only the content of the essay, but the competence and skill of whichever editor approved its publication. My righteous feminist tirade was completely unchecked in tone or in consideration of my audience. When I reread the thing months later, when I was off hormones, I was shocked at my inappropriate and unbridled criticism of people well above my head. I'm usually far too professionally savvy to make such an egregious misstep.

This email bit me in the butt in a big way. I was called into a mandatory meeting with the editor-in-chief, the writer of the essay, and the editor who approved the op-ed. I asked to have a union representative or my manager with me in the meeting but was refused. The three women tag-teamed me, verbally scolding and shaming me for the email in a humiliating half-hour video conference. It was horrible.

Lesson learned. You may not be yourself on all these hormones. I certainly wasn't.

Other than the fallout of my emotionally overwrought performance at work, I actually loved the ritual of the injections. Yeah, it was scary at first. But here I was shoving more than five thousand dollars' worth of drugs in my body. Surely this would be the answer? It felt like I was doing the most concrete thing yet to make a baby happen. It was extreme, and I was ready to get extreme.

Dr. Patronizing told me that he saw what looked like five or six eggs growing incrementally each time I came in to be monitored. I dutifully continued my routine, waiting for the day when

I could finally have the procedure and find out how many of those little eggs were retrieved.

But here's the thing about IVF that I didn't know yet: It's a game of attrition. With every step you tend to lose some ground. Let me explain. Let's say you're a healthy thirty-five-year-old and your doctor gets ten eggs from your retrieval. The next step is to fertilize those eggs. Well, maybe only nine of those eggs are mature, and just seven of them are actually fertilized. Then they have to grow for five days until they reach a level of cellular complexity known as the blastocyst phase. Many embryos stop growing and developing before then, so perhaps five of those embryos actually make it to the blast stage. Next, it's time to send those out for genetic testing. One to three weeks later you may find out only two or three of those embryos are genetically healthy and normal.

Every step of the way you lose ground. Therefore, the first number—how many eggs you get—is so important.

This explanation is an oversimplification, of course. There are many other variations in the steps that can occur, depending on what your doctor calls for and what options you choose.

In the past, clinics would put the sperm in a petri dish with an egg, and let it find its way to fertilization. These days it's more common (for an added price, of course) for doctors to recommend ICSI, or intracytoplasmic sperm injection. This just means they inject the sperm directly into the egg to encourage fertilization.

If all goes to plan, the sperm and egg unite and start to divide into multiple cells. By day five—or even three—some people choose to transfer fresh embryos, but multiple studies have found greater success with transferring embryos that were first frozen. No one knows why.

It had been strange explaining this whole situation to the people in my life, who at the time were mostly the neighbors who shared my backyard paradise. Throughout the pandemic we kept each other sane while staying socially distant. One day, shortly after a home insemination with The Lawyer (just before starting IVF), I tried to explain the nuance of the whole procedure to several of my neighbors as we enjoyed the warm fall weather and shared some snacks in the backyard. We sat in a semicircle of mismatched lawn furniture around two adjacent outdoor tables.

"I need to understand. Please, from the beginning, you have this sperm donor? And what happens?" asked Rita, a fifty-nine-year-old chain-smoking Lebanese woman who owned the bodega around the corner and made killer tabbouleh. She was everyone's mother-by-proxy in the backyard. Rita fed us and looked out for us, and generally looked beautiful and ageless, except for the occasional white roots that crept up around her forehead.

"The sperm donor lives a reasonable distance away," I explained. "I take the Metro about half an hour and then I will be meeting him at an apartment, and on the second floor there's an office space in the building, and there's public restrooms there. The donor's going to deposit a, um, sample into a menstrual cup."

"Why doesn't he do it directly?" Rita said, her accent accompanied by a hand motion to indicate sex.

Ashley, another neighbor, suppressed a laugh and ran her hand through her short blond hair while giving me an amused, meaningful look. Ashley is an undeniably stunning thirty-seven-year-old woman with a killer smile, sparkling green eyes, and a phenomenal sense of style. Plus, her nonjudgmental attitude had a way of making people feel included in things—as if you and she were the only ones in on a private joke.

"He has a fiancée," I explained. It seemed simpler to leave it at that.

"So, he's not having sex with Valerie to make this baby, he's just providing sperm," Ashley added, making eye contact with me to confirm that I approved of her explanation.

"Okay," Rita said, still looking suspicious.

"He's just a donor," I said. "And remember how things got complicated before, when I slept with that other sperm donor?"

Rita waved her hands, dismissing any talk of The Conquistador—who did not have a very good reputation in these parts.

"Do you take it and go home?" Rita asked, adding: "Eat something," as she pushed a small bowl of almonds across the table toward me.

"No, no. I go in the bathroom. Immediately insert it using a menstrual cup that rests against my cervix. And then I take the train home and cross my fingers."

"I know sperm lives for five days," Rita said. "What I'm worried about is that it won't reach."

"Right," said Jo, Ashley's sister and roommate. "Because the menstrual cup doesn't get up that far."

"It gets the sperm pretty close," I said. "There are two kinds. One sits in your vaginal canal. The other one slides in and pops over the donut-shaped cervix and holds the sperm right against the cervix. That's the kind that I use."

Jo and Rita nodded and murmured words of understanding. Jo, a mom to a fantastic eighteen-year-old, was the first single mom I approached to ask for advice about my whole plan to be a solo parent. In addition to having a dimple-cheekbone combo that could make you weep, Jo is a pillar of the D.C. lesbian community, and co-owner of the iconic As You Are bar in Capitol Hill. From the beginning, she was incredibly supportive of my unorthodox efforts to have a child.

"How long do you leave it in?" Jo asked. "And sit with your feet up?"

"You can leave it in up to twelve hours," I said. "But lie down on my back? Not long, because I have to take the Metro home first anyway. And the sperm know where to go."

"You're ovulating right this moment?" Ashley asked.

"Well, I should be ovulating in a day or two. My first insemination was day before yesterday. And it was really strange. He went in the bathroom and produced it and I went in this kind of public restroom and you know, basically inserted it and wow, I guess this is what single women have to do."

"Your experience has so many levels," Jo said. "I'm going to ask you a personal question. Have you masturbated of late? Like, is there fluid happening for you?" She turned to Rita and Ashley before explaining: "My first piece of advice to Valerie for getting pregnant was to masturbate a lot. Like, really get in touch with your body."

"I have. I will say, this morning, the fluid was, well, I wasn't expecting so much! But I wiped after going to the bathroom, and it was dripping off the tissue and looked like egg whites. Which is exactly what you want."

"Yeah," Jo agreed. "I think there is actual scientific conversation surrounding the more lubricated the female body is the more successful your chances are likely to be."

"Because the vaginal canal can be hostile for sperm," I added. "It's the female fluid that makes it survivable."

I really appreciated their curiosity and the way these women encouraged me to keep my head up, even when I felt hopeless about getting pregnant.

"You have people surrounding you and coddling you with love and lifting you up. You have our support," Jo said.

"I know," I said, a little catch in my voice. "It's like a little nest of positivity around here."

"So, go get some sperm!" Rita said, causing everyone to laugh.

AFTER WEEKS OF STICKING MYSELF with needles, I was ready for them to put me under and use their very narrow needle to extract any eggs I'd produced. Dr. Patronizing had been seeing about five or six follicles at my monitoring appointments, so I was hopeful that I would at least get that many eggs. It wasn't a ton of eggs—younger women can retrieve dozens. Still, for my age, things were looking pretty good.

I was so excited the night before that I could barely sleep. It felt like Christmas Eve as a kid. I'd been to acupuncture earlier in the afternoon, drank my herbs, taken the supplements, and did my final trigger injection—which sends the signal to the ovaries to release the eggs so they can begin the journey down the fallopian tubes and toward the uterus.

I lay in bed comically early (I popped melatonin at eight p.m. because I just wanted to go to sleep and get on with it already) with my hands crossed on my lower abdomen. I inhaled and exhaled, concentrating and slowing my breath as I silently chanted my mantra: *I am the mother; I am the child.*

I woke up and was basically levitating around my apartment with anticipation as I prepared for the clinic.

I arrived early, and everything went smoothly. They had me change into a surgery gown and wear a hairnet-like cap. As I drifted off to sleep, I tried to ask how soon I would find out about how many eggs they were able to get. I lost consciousness before getting an answer.

When I awoke, I had a Post-it stuck to my left hand. It had the number three with a circle around it.

"No," I thought, still groggy from anesthesia. "There must have been more than three! This can't be how they tell me . . . ?"

It was, though. That's how they communicated that they had only retrieved three eggs, with only one looking (barely) mature enough to be fertilized. Finally, after at least twenty or thirty minutes, the doctor materialized. When I tried to ask why things had gone so wrong, he gruffly said the outcome was exactly what he expected.

Still fuzzy-headed, I asked him why, in that case, had he told me before the procedure to anticipate five or six eggs, instead of setting my own expectations more realistically. Visibly annoyed, Dr. Patronizing blamed me.

"You're almost forty and you have old eggs," he barked. "It's not my fault!" I was stunned by this last bit, which had the ring of a five-year-old denying he was the one who wiped a booger on the wall.

Dr. Patronizing turned on his heel and marched away, leaving me alone, stunned and grieving. I was shocked at his defensiveness. I knew my body was failing. I knew I was the problem. But he failed me, too. He should have talked to me about realistic outcomes. Instead, everything up to this point had felt like a never-ending sales pitch about his unrivaled thirty-four years of experience getting people pregnant. That bravado was nowhere to be found on my egg retrieval day.

The next afternoon, a nurse from the clinic called to unceremoniously tell me that none of my eggs had fertilized. The doctor usually makes this phone call, but mine didn't bother. I couldn't believe the cycle was a complete bust. Not a single embryo. No blasts to test for genetic abnormalities. No babies for me.

I went home and climbed into my bed. And the gray came and settled in on me like a dense fog.

"The gray" is my name for the depression I've been trying to outrun my whole life. I manage my mental health very well, and with the support of family, friends, and a good therapist. But this . . . I couldn't outrun this.

This whole process had stretched on for so long now. I had been trying, and putting one foot in front of the other without letting disappointment creep in. It was too much now.

I hadn't done any drinking in months because I was detoxing for fertility purposes. Now I bought a big bottle of Jameson, grabbed a coffee mug, and got into bed with both. I poured, I sipped, I slept, I woke, I cried, I sipped. I called in sick to work on Monday. I went back Tuesday but was barely functional.

To be honest, all I wanted was my fucking mommy. But that was out of the question. I'd kept this entire process secret from her for over a year at this point and couldn't begin to picture how to break the news to her.

Complicating things, she was coming out to visit before the end of the week—timing I didn't fully think through. Still raw from the disappointment, I feared I would break down and tell her everything. She knows me incredibly well and could already tell I was off whenever we spoke—which was almost every day.

"I'm so excited to see you!" she cooed into the phone just before getting on the plane.

"Yeah, me too, Mom." I could tell I wasn't mustering the appropriate level of enthusiasm.

"What's wrong?"

"Nothing, Mom. I'm just tired. It's going to be so great to see you. Really."

I knew her momma-sense was tingling, but I was determined to keep my baby plans under wraps. This was a woman who had talked me out of three tattoos. There was no way I was going to give her the opportunity to exercise her impressive level of influence on something so important to me.

I was still thrilled and relieved to see her. I hugged her for probably a weirdly long time on the street of row houses, in front of my brick apartment building with the bright red door. There's just something about your mom's warmth and smell when you're feeling down in the dumps. It's comfort. Home.

I could tell she was keeping an extra close eye on me as we hung out, watching *Catfish* while doing our makeup and giggling at the absurdity of the reality show. We walked together on my usual four-mile morning route down to the Navy Yard and the Anacostia River, then up through Southeast Capitol Hill to the Northeast part, until we were almost to H Street before looping back home. We went out to expensive restaurants the first few nights and I got up the courage to broach the possibility of pursuing the foster-to-adopt path. During my fog in the immediate days after the failed egg retrieval I had delved into the options in my own community and started filling out paperwork to start the training process. I had always had an interest in fostering. I just thought it would happen later, after I had some kids the old-fashioned way.

My mom was surprisingly supportive of the idea of fostering. The idea of a single mother was less offensive to her when the children already had no one. She even came with me to view a few two- and three-bedroom apartments—just in case I decided to go down that path. Just discussing this possibility and trying to envision a future of becoming a mother (one way or another) was a soothing thought. It felt good to share this little piece of my vision with my mom.

Ultimately, I wasn't able to keep it from her.

It happened in her rental car. She was driving us to a little town in Virginia for a girls' day of shopping and coffee and fun. About thirty minutes into the ride, I broke down crying.

"Mom?" I said, between sobs. "I've got to tell you something."

Clearly alarmed, my mom kept her eyes mostly on the road, with a few sideways glances darted my way.

"Okay . . ."

"Mom, what would you do if one of your kids was gay?"

Now, this may seem like a counterintuitive opening. But keep in mind my parents are extremely Catholic, and being gay is still not accepted in the Church. I hadn't really thought this line of questioning through, but I had a point: I was trying to ask about her capacity for accepting her children as they were, despite the religious and cultural taboos to which my parents clung.

"I . . . would try to support them and accept them as they were," my mom said, with barely a lick of hesitation.

Stunned, this was all I needed to hear to open the flood-gates of words that had been beating against the inside of my mouth.

As the tears and sentences poured out of my body, my mother—an utter superhero—just gripped the steering wheel with one hand and reached over with her other to pat my knee and hold my hand. And she listened.

"I've . . . I've been trying to have a baby, to become a single mother by choice with donor sperm for over a year now . . ."

Her eyes widened, but she kept listening, occasionally whispering, "It's okay," in hushed, soothing tones.

Whenever I paused in my confession, she would pat my knee and say, "Valerie, I'm here. I'm right here for you. I love you. I just have to keep my eyes on the road right now, traffic is a little hairy, but I'm right here."

"Wait, Mom, there's more . . ." I had to pause in between heaves. "I found a sperm donor on Facebook, so I was doing home insemination with a guy I just met online . . . I know it sounds crazy . . . but there's more. I just went through IVF, and I've been on all these hormones for so long, and . . . Mom! It didn't work. I spent all this money, and I may never have a baby."

I paused to let a few sobs escape at this point.

"Okay—" my mom started.

"Wait, Mom, there's more . . . I'm writing a book about this whole journey and I'm going to go public with it. So, everyone is going to know . . ."

I think I stopped to blow my nose when she finally had a chance to speak.

"You know how I feel about this," she said. "But I would never want one of my kids to not live their life the way they wanted to because they were afraid of what I would think."

Those words were like a magical incantation that instantly broke a lifelong spell. I was stunned into silence, barring a few residual sniffs and blowing of my nose. My mom really did love me unconditionally, and she was capable of supporting me, emotionally, in exactly the way I had hoped—the way I had needed her to be there for me. I could live my life—be myself out loud—without fear of losing her love and acceptance.

The calm that settled over me was overwhelming. It was utter peace. For the first time in a long time, I let go of the constant baby worries and just let my body and soul unclench. We spent the rest of the day drinking too much coffee and picking out a birdhouse for my backyard before driving back to D.C.

It was a good thing that the news went over as well as it did. My next IVF cycle was about to start.

This time I had my mom in my corner.

Chapter Thirteen
The Man

AFTER MONTHS OF HORMONES, ABSTAINING from booze and focusing on being the healthiest vessel I could be for my hypothetical baby, I was in the mood for something different: to actually be different—more myself.

I wanted to feel like a woman. I wanted to be desired. I wanted to go on a date.

It was strange to make the transition from the Facebook groups and Just a Baby app to the world of online dating. The two worlds felt similar, but sperm people were just more direct about what they wanted. As I swiped, I made a wish to meet someone for whom I could feel even a glimmer of a spark.

I was not prepared for what came next.

The very first date I went on, I met him. The Man. And, well, The Man changed everything.

Even before we met, we talked over video chat for *four freaking hours*. I quickly discovered he was exactly my type: tall, smart, and masculine as hell. He was a man's man who could fix cars, rewire the electricity in your house, or redo your plumbing.

He would be clutch in a zombie apocalypse.

I walked into the bar and instantly spotted his bearded grin, and suddenly, this teddy bear of a human was walking toward me and shaking my hand. I eyed the gap in his teeth, his dimples, and the gray hairs sprouting among the black curls on his head, and I knew I wanted him.

I'm going to make this man fall in love with me, I immediately thought, naively assuming he was the only one about to be swept off their feet.

We had a beer, but left right after, because they didn't have Jameson and I'm not a beer drinker. He was mildly amused and a good sport about this as we made our way down the street.

Most of what came next was a blur. We sat down at an Irish spot, and he told me about his military service. An army brat myself, I have great respect and gratitude for those who served, and he seemed to appreciate that. I don't know what came over me, but at some point during the evening, I raised a glass of whiskey and offered up a toast to my "spectacular rack." He laughed his big, open laugh, because this, to him, was hilarious. He would later remind me of this moment in front of other people, much to my embarrassment.

As the night wore on, I decided to let him give me a ride home. Something about The Man made me feel safe and taken care of. He radiated warmth. I boldly invited him for a nightcap in my backyard. It was June and late enough that the mosquitoes had finally gone to bed, but the air was still humid, embracing our bare legs in its thick warmth.

We sat down across from each other and smiled nervously, now out of the noisy bar and away from the energy of dozens of other drunk patrons . . . it was just us and the moonlight. Staring into each other's eyes, like a couple of nerds.

And then he leaned over and kissed me.

My God, he kissed me like we were both dying tomorrow. I felt the rest of my body drift away and my whole being, my whole self had become no more than the beating heart of my lips against his. When we parted, I kept my eyes closed and head tilted back, dazed, still drunk on him, floating in the moment. When I opened them, I saw his eyes were closed, too—just for split second—before he blinked and smiled at me. This wasn't a spark. This was nuclear fusion.

I bridged the space between us and crawled onto his lap. I straddled his legs and started to devour him (this is where my nickname, Spidermonkey, eventually came from). I ran my hands through his hair as he pulled me closer in his arms and held me tight. I felt my body melt into his; we were moving in unison, gently rocking back and forth, chasing each other's lips, our hands everywhere. He occasionally paused to pull my head back, gaze into my eyes, and stroke my hair as I held his face between my hands. And then the kissing, spurred by the magnetic pull of two forces irresistibly drawn to each other, would begin again. The chemistry was unreal.

Finally, he had to go home. It was three a.m. and we both had to work in the morning. It was a fucking Tuesday night. I walked him to his car and watched as he drove away, revving his engine as he left.

As I fell asleep that night I touched my fingertips gently against my lips, still electric and puffy from all their clandestine evening activities, and I wondered when I would see this man, The Man, again.

For the first time in over a year, I wanted something other than a baby. The Man had—somehow—made me forget for a few magical hours about my tragic routine of peeing on ovulation sticks, poking myself with needles, and the constant ever-loving yearning to be a mother. He made me feel like more than a defective womb.

I fell asleep, still smelling him on my clothes.

"Good morning, beautiful."

I was stunned. He had texted me by eight a.m. the very next day. That doesn't happen. I wasn't sure how to react. This was unprecedented.

Our second date was at a Balkan restaurant on D.C.'s Barracks Row. He beamed at me from across the table, an open book, unafraid to tell me pretty much everything he was thinking and feeling.

And then he asked me: "Do you want to have kids?"

I froze, but before I could say anything, he proudly announced: "I had a vasectomy!"

I cleared my throat, obviously uncomfortable, and the cheeky grin evaporated from his face.

"Um, that's complicated. Can we get into it another time?"

"Sure, of course." He smiled apologetically and explained that he had two grown children, his first born when he was still a teenager. He had the vasectomy after the second, because he had lost so much of his youth to parenting and knew he wanted independence in his forties.

I took this information in and quietly tried to accept that this might not work out. I mean, he was a good kisser, but it was date two—what did I expect? I was injecting myself with hormones twice a day, for Christ's sake. I had another egg retrieval coming up. I had to keep my eye on the prize.

But those dimples . . . and the way he looked at me with that wide-open facial expression. The Man wore no mask. He wanted me to see the real him. As we walked through D.C. that night, fingers linked, he slowly started showing me all his wounds—and not just the missing tip of his ring finger, lost in a motorcycle accident. I felt like I knew him my whole life. He unfolded for me, like a letter from an old friend, careworn from the familiarity of words reread too many times to count. He told me of his childhood hurts, the heartaches and moments of emptiness. His bleakest moments.

"I can't believe how much I'm sharing with you. I don't do this," he said. "It just feels so easy with you."

His words had the tingly effect that I'm told ASMR videos are supposed to create, starting at the nape of my neck and climbing slowly across my scalp with electric anticipation.

That night, I contemplated just breaking things off without an explanation. But some part of me had hope. I was going to have to tell The Man about my baby plans. Like, immediately. Before date three.

He called me the next night; we had already started speaking in the evenings, for hours at a time, even falling asleep on the phone together.

"I need to tell you something," I started.

"Uh-oh . . ." He chuckled halfheartedly. "Should I be worried?"

"This isn't easy," I said. "And you might not want to see me anymore when I tell you. But I'm just going to say it."

"Okay," he said, patiently.

"I . . . I have been going through IVF and trying to get pregnant."

"Oh?

I could tell I was about to machine-gun-fire the words out of my mouth.

"So, it's a little weird. Am I doing this? I'm doing this. So, I'm actually working on a huge project to tell the story of my journey trying to become a mom. I've been working with a sperm donor I found on Facebook, which sounds crazy—I mean, it is crazy, like home insemination—Hello? Who am I, right? But it's not as bad as it sounds, it's not like I'm doing natural insemination, ha. Except The Conquistador, but he doesn't count. Er, no, what I mean is, I had him—the donor—get all the tests and everything, so it's all aboveboard. Except I did have to lie to my doctor. Which I shouldn't have had to, I mean, ha, do you have any idea how vague federal law is about defining a sexually intimate partner? Anyway, I don't even know if it's going to work. I mean, for a while now, my whole life has been about cervical fluid, counting follicles, and tracking my ovulation. I just did one egg retrieval and got zero embryos. Now I'm getting ready for another, but there's no guarantee that it will even happen. So, I'm totally, probably not going to have a baby. But I hope it does work. I definitely want a baby. So, there's that. I'll shut up now. Are you freaked out? You're totally freaked out, aren't you?"

The Man paused. And then he surprised me.

"I really like you . . . I, no. I'm not scared away by that. I mean, I have questions—uh, The Conquistador? But it doesn't change how I feel about you. I haven't felt like this in a long time."

I melted. Into a puddle. I think he kept talking, but I have no idea what he said, because my brain was setting off fireworks and my insides went all warm and fuzzy. I muted the phone and did a happy dance. I squeezed my eyes shut—so tight—and crossed my fingers and told the universe I would do anything if she could just let me have this new vision of my future that had just materialized before my eyes.

Could I finally get everything? A baby? A man? A family?

Inconceivable

. . .

WE COULDN'T STAY APART.

Day after day, he would drive to my apartment after work, we would drink each other in until falling asleep, tangled in each other's limbs. And then The Man would crawl out of my bed at five thirty in the morning to go to work, an hour away. I spent every minute of every weekend at his place.

These early days were magic. We couldn't get enough of each other. He made me laugh. He made me dance, one arm around my waist and the other holding my hand as we swayed around my tiny kitchen while the Commodores crooned "Easy Like Sunday Morning." I made him brisket in my shitty oven— and he was actually blown away.

He was making me start to believe that maybe I was somebody who could fall in love and be loved back. It sounds achingly simple as I type it, but I had twenty years of bad dates behind me. I had already grieved never finding exactly what appeared to be right in front of me, right now. It was disorienting. It had been ten years since the one time I was truly in love. Now thirty-nine, I had given up on the dream of a partner, and found true peace and happiness as a single person. The Man disrupted my entire sense of reality. Every day he got better, and kinder. Every day he asked me to just keep communicating with him so we could always make things work and be this happy together. He awoke something in me that had been dead so long that I had forgotten it had ever existed. Somewhere in the back of my head, I was trying to sort out this new contradiction to my long-established foregone conclusion that I would never again fall in love. The Man was making a believer out of me.

Two weeks after meeting him, we were lying in bed at his house, my head in the crook of his arm as I absentmindedly swirled his little cyclone of curly chest hair around my index finger. The Man looked at me with a grin, pointed to the door behind my head, and said: "That room would make a great nursery."

Three weeks after meeting him, he told me he loved me. With zero hesitation, I said it back.

I was romantic, too. I found a book of postcards with romance novel covers on them in a pile of free stuff during one of my walks through Capitol Hill. I wrote him little love notes on the backs of each one and hid them everywhere around his house. He delighted each time he found one—say in the freezer, in the side door of his car, or in the pocket of a jacket he hadn't worn in ages.

We hated being apart to an irrational degree, and I hated seeing how tired he was driving to and from my house all the time. Early on he asked me to stay with him at his house in the woods, about an hour outside of D.C. For a week.

"What about my cats?" (I had two.)

"I love cats. Bring them."

"What!?"

He shrugged and smiled that open, genuine smile. My heart expanded like an accordion and I let out a little sigh.

He really loves me.

We transported two cats, a litter box, a scratching post, and cat food to his place, and basically played house for the week.

My mom was initially thrilled when I told her I had met the man I was going to marry. I had never said anything close to this to my mom before, and she was (understandably) very excited.

Then she said: "Why are you whispering?"

"Momma, I'm at his house . . . I'm staying with him for the week."

The words hung in the air as my mom let this sink in.

"Valerie! Don't you move in with him!" She was laughing, but I could tell her concern was genuine.

"Mom, I'm obviously not going to move in with him. Definitely not. It's just for the week. I gotta go, okay?"

THE MAN CONTINUED TO SUPPORT my baby dreams. He injected me with my IVF hormones. He drove me to my egg retrieval and wiped away my tears when I got five eggs. And then three embryos. Finally, when genetic testing came back, I learned that I had two healthy embryos—one girl and one boy.

At one point we were both sitting in his massive bathtub, and he offered to have his sperm checked to see if they were still viable via an invasive procedure. He took off his glasses, rubbed his face, and looked at me earnestly, eyes wide open, and said that even though he'd had a vasectomy, he was open to having the doctor attempt to extract any sperm he may have so that the child I had could be his.

My heart swelled when he said this. I was a bit in shock. After my experience with The Conquistador, I was a bit gun shy about sharing my child with someone I hadn't known for very long. I told him that I would have to think about it. We never ended up exploring this option, but it gave me even more faith that he was supportive of my plans to become a mother.

Two months into this unyielding romance, The Man asked me to move in with him. Even though this meant I would be leaving behind the city and friends I loved, I agreed and packed my things up to start a new life with him in the woods. We had known each other only three months, but we both kept telling everyone: "When you know, you know."

We were approaching forty. We should know what we were doing. Whatever happened, we were in it together.

Even so, something slowly started shifting. It was barely perceptible, but just below the surface, I could feel it. He was off. We were off. It was two weeks before we moved in together that I had a terrible sense that it must be about the baby.

I had already told The Man at this point that I may wait to move forward with transferring an embryo and getting pregnant to give us a little more time to grow in our relationship. Once I had two embryos on ice, I was able to relax a bit about my ticking clock. Early on we had talked about parenting together, and how important it was for both people to back each other up on issues, particularly discipline. We seemed to have similar ideals, but more recently he hadn't been as enthusiastic about those conversations, and he was quick to cling to the idea of putting off the baby. With the move fast approaching, I tried to broach the subject again.

"I'm trying to figure out when would be a good time to transfer an embryo. I mean, it would be great to give us another six months to a year, what do you think? What's the sweet spot?"

We were driving in his car through winding roads in the woods near his house. I loved these drives, because I'm a speed junky and he had souped up his engine so it roared as he flew down the curving paths, windows rolled down.

"Honestly, there is no sweet spot," he said, instantly worrying me. "There's never really a good time for it."

I was silent after he said this. My entire apartment was already in boxes, and I had given notice to my building manager. His answer was the opposite of what I had hoped to hear.

It was hard for me to reconcile this occasional coldness that he would exhibit with the usual version of him that was so warm, sweet, and wonderful. Whenever the gray threatened to take over, The Man would smile that wide-open smile and hold me against his chest, let me bury my head in him until my worst thoughts went away. No one had ever made me feel so safe. Besides, I had made it clear to him that I was definitely going to need to become a mom, one way or another. That wasn't negotiable.

He knew that! I was clear from the start. He wouldn't ask me to give that up.

My ticket had been punched and the ride had taken off before I was fully strapped in. All I could do was push the feelings of doubt deep into my subconscious and try to reassure myself that The Man would never take my dream away from me.

But the lack of answers began to wear on me. His older sister came into town for a short visit just before the move. She was wonderful—we hit it off immediately. But I had a panic attack in the middle of her trip because I could see the way The Man grew quiet when I talked about my baby plans with her. I inadvertently started crying, alone in his bedroom. He came looking for me, found me, took me in his arms, and asked: "What's wrong?"

"I'm afraid you don't want me to have a baby and I'm scared what that means," I said in between my sobs. He hadn't seen me like this, at my most emotionally strung out. "I really want to know right now if you're changing your mind about the baby thing."

He held me, but then gently chided me for "doing this" while his sister was in town and said he couldn't give me an answer about the baby right there, right then. Which—fair. But I was about to give up everything I had for this vision of a life that he had promised me. I couldn't help that my nervous breakdown was happening when an out-of-town guest was present.

I wanted him to reassure me that nothing had changed. He couldn't, or wouldn't, do that. Instead, he said it wasn't the right time to discuss it.

"I'm about to move in with you," I implored, a bit too passively for even my own liking.

He said it was too big a topic to get into with family in town, and insisted we go back downstairs to his sister.

Denial is incredibly powerful. Every day I put one foot in front of the other, until suddenly I was moving into The Man's massive house in the middle of nowhere. It was a big adjustment for this admitted city girl. But in a hundred different ways, living together was instant bliss. We began the delightful task of nesting together. He had lived in his four-bedroom, three-bathroom house for less than a year and had hardly any decorations on the walls. He let me put up some of my art—though not all. My taste was far more eclectic than his. But he kept stressing that he wanted me to feel like it was my home too. And it gradually started to feel that way.

"I'm going to spoil you," he said.

I had this wonderful man who came home to me every night. And that's all I wanted from him. I, after working a full day from home, would run to greet him at the door, where he would wrap me in his arms and kiss me deeply until my head went to that faraway place that I discovered the first night our lips met. Sometimes he would sneak in and scare me as a prank—jumping out and shouting "BOO!" To which I would inevitably respond with a jump and a shriek, and then we would giggle and chase each other around the house.

Then, just two and a half weeks after I moved in, The Man came home from work and asked me to sit down on the couch with him.

"We need to talk." Between his choice of words and the serious, closed facial expression he was wearing, I was afraid he was breaking up with me. I knew it in my bones. It was over.

The Man

None of this was real. No man will ever love me, or stay. Oh God, please don't leave me.

I couldn't help the intrusive thoughts, but tried to push them aside as we sat down on the wraparound couch in his living room. The house was on the edge of a forest preserve, outside of D.C. It had huge windows that splashed a palette of greens and blues from every wall, thanks to the surrounding trees and seemingly endless blue skies. I felt my vulnerability acutely as I stared out into the woods, toward the spot where deer would approach the edge of his property, eyeing us nervously until we came out to feed them.

In this moment, my heart was his to smash.

"I can't be with someone who is having a baby."

The words echoed through my head. He kept talking in that serious, low voice. He sounded very sorry. The thing was, he had realized that he didn't want another baby or a child in his life. He couldn't be a parent again. He had his first child after accidentally getting a girl pregnant as a teenager. He married her and spent two decades raising children who were now adults, sacrificing everything (as parents do).

Now, he realized, was his time to finally be free from those responsibilities. He couldn't be with a partner who was raising an infant because there was no way he wouldn't become deeply involved in that child's life. He was afraid to fall in love with a child that I was technically having with another man; I could take that baby away from him at any time. The alternative was for him to adopt the child—which could leave him paying child

support if we were to later break up. It was impossibly complicated and emotional.

His words flattened me. I thought I was building a life with
this man, but I had just been stacking buckets of sand—like an
asshole—too close to the coming tide.

I could feel my face had gone slack, except for my eyes,
which were wide open, bulging and taut, from the tears I was
holding back. I wanted to cry. I wanted to scream.

*This would have been useful information a month ago! How could
you do this? Did you trap me here on purpose?*

I should have said: *Who even are you? Where is The Man I fell
in love with?*

Instead, I said: "Are you breaking up with me?"

That was it. In a small, little girl voice, I asked him this
stupid question. I apologized to myself inwardly for being this
weak. For betraying the baby who I knew I needed to have.
But in this moment, I was choosing him.

His furrowed brow relaxed into a cautious smile when he
heard my whispered voice.

He shook his head: "No."

He scooped me into his lap and brushed the hair out of
my eyes.

"No." He kissed me. "I just know myself and know that
I'm not going to change my mind."

The anger flared in me, bright for a moment. And then he
touched my cheek. The fire was extinguished.

"I want to be with you forever," I said. It wasn't a lie.

"I want to be with you forever," he answered.

He pulled me into his chest, where I nestled and closed my eyes and willed myself to be numb.

At least you have him. Give it some time. You can figure this out.

Thus began a daily battle in which I pitted my undeniable love for this man against what I knew I had to do to be true to myself. I wouldn't know it right away, but I would never be able to fully trust him again after he put me through this bait-and-switch. It was a rapid erosion of the complete trust I had put in him. It was also the very first moment I stopped being fully honest with him. For the first time in this relationship, my true feelings were now secrets that I had to keep.

As much as it pained me, on a certain level I understood where The Man was coming from. Not that what he did wasn't fucked up. Because it was.

Up until this point (an admittedly short period of time) I had seen him as an incredibly unselfish person. As he told it, he had put other people's needs ahead of him for his entire adult life, joining the military at nineteen, going to war. He wanted to travel on his own terms, pursue his dream career without other obligations. He wanted to live the life—frankly—that I had led up until now. I had traveled and pursued my dreams and partied and lived free of major responsibility for my entire adult life. I was ready for the anchor of a child and a family. We were in fundamentally different places, but so completely in love.

I can't explain it. And I was so angry with myself—so angry—but I couldn't walk away from him. I comforted myself

with the thought of my two embryos. I could pursue this relationship. Hope he would soften and change his mind. Or see if
I could be happy enough with just him.

*Anything but leaving him. I can't, I can't, I can't. Not yet. Maybe
not ever.*

I knew my internal equivocating was also unfair to him. I
rushed face-first into this love affair. I wanted to see it through.

And then things shifted again. It started slowly. It was barely
noticeable, the way relationship quicksand finds its way into your
home. At first it just swallows your ankles. "I'm fine," you think,
kicking it aside as you traverse the kitchen. Then, suddenly,
you're vacuuming the living room and it's up to your waist. "I'm
happy," you insist as you breathe your last gasp before the sand
completely overtakes you. And then you're just gone.

I noticed the way he picked at me first. Sometimes he played
it off like he was just observing things about me. But it always
came off as critical.

"That's how you brush your teeth!?" he asked one night,
incredulous and horrified as he watched me preparing for bed.
I froze, my toothbrush still jammed against my cheek. I eyed
myself and quickly spit in the sink, rinsed my mouth, and spit
again. We made eye contact in the mirror, and he just laughed
like he was being silly. But after he left the bathroom, I wiped
my mouth on my towel self-consciously; something about his
tone had given life to a brand-new insecurity—about this really
weird, specific thing. It grabbed me by the throat every time he
critiqued my actions or asked me to explain my rationale for the

way I did something. I had lived alone for most of my adult life. I wasn't used to being observed.

Another day, he stood behind me as I washed the dishes and started telling me I was doing it wrong and wasting the water by letting it run. I think he was probably right, but as a lifelong renter whose mom taught her to wash the dishes many moons ago . . . it genuinely hadn't occurred to me. And I thought I had it covered. Frustrated, I asked, "Do you want to do it?"

"Fine!" he said, his voice thin and tight.

I turned off the water and left the kitchen.

It got worse. After a few more months he started turning me down for sex and being less affectionate.

"Can I snuggle you?" I asked, as I usually did, one night as we turned on the TV and prepared to sink into the couch.

"No." He crossed the room, sat on the other couch, and looked at me, blank. His face was closed off, eyes cold. "I don't feel like it right now."

I'm all for consent. But he was so needlessly icy and dismissive. He knew this hurt me. It would have cost him nothing to say the exact same thing more gently. But he couldn't seem to afford to do that, for some reason.

I developed an addiction to lingerie, thinking I could lure the old him, the warm him, back to me. But the confident version of myself, who didn't even wonder stupid things, like whether she was sexy—that Valerie was fucking disappearing.

In between these moments were a hundred other good, happy ones that made it easier for me to justify staying.

We took a road trip over Thanksgiving, seeing several friends and loved ones along the way. He held my hand for most of the trip. Whenever I reached across the car to caress his face, he would immediately reciprocate by leaning his cheek into my hand, again gazing at me with that wide-open face, and it felt like I could maybe make this work. That maybe he would be enough for me.

We slept in a Vermont sugarhouse that fall—one of the little wooden huts where they collect and process maple syrup. We also headed to Upstate New York and stayed next door to my first apartment in Albany on State Street—just blocks from the state capitol, where I had previously covered politics from my office for the Associated Press. We also made it to Boston that November, where another one of my friends from the Albany days made us an obscene Thanksgiving feast.

We spent Christmas with his sister, brother-in-law, and niece. They opened their whole hearts to me, and I loved them and dreamed of being a part of this welcoming, happy family. I had glimpses of what a happy life could be like with him, long-term. What guarantee was there that my embryos were going to be successful anyway? I had this wonderful man right in front of me. He was real and tangible, and he smelled so fucking good, and I just wanted to be able to bite his lower lip, just a little bit. Every day. For the rest of my life, please.

I can't stress this enough: I was part of a couple. Someone had chosen me. I wasn't alone. For the first time since my heart was smashed three weeks before my thirtieth birthday, the exact thing I had grieved not having, the thing I had worked so hard to let go of wanting . . . I fucking had it. A partner.

Wasn't that so much better than an imaginary baby? Sure, right now it was a perfect dream baby that promised to grow up into a delightful Gilmore Girl of a child who would rapid-fire pop culture or literary references and eat pounds of junk food without ever gaining more than a tummy-ache.

What if this kid actually turns out to be terrible?

The Man is a known quantity. The baby could be an asshole.

These were the things I bargained with myself over. The Man loved me in exactly the way I needed to be loved. Most of the time. Then less of the time. Eventually hardly at all.

Those thin walls made of unspoken frustrations and silent contempt started erecting themselves between us. At night we no longer slept in an ergonomically correct, double-pretzel configuration. We would chastely kiss goodnight before rolling over to face away from each other for the evening.

"Butt to butt," we'd say, snickering, as we assumed the position.

It was the same position I would lie in for hours each night, frozen, afraid to wake him behind me. I would scroll through videos on YouTube from various psychologists and psychiatrists unpacking my unspoken insecurities about the relationship.

Actual YouTube videos I have watched or saved to watch later (it started innocently enough):

"10 Ways to Heal Abandonment Trauma"

"9 Reasons Why You Feel So Lonely"

"8 Signs You Were Actually in Love"

Then the recommendations got darker, and more on the nose:

"Do Not Love Half Lovers"

"7 Signs They're Not the One"

"Toxic Relationships: How to Leave in 7 Steps"

I knew something wasn't right. I could feel it in my gut. I couldn't admit it to myself, and certainly not to him . . . but I would never forgive him for the baby thing. I wasn't mad. I was broken. I gave him an out when I told him about my plans before date three. How could he put me in this impossible position?

And if he had to, why did he have to stop loving me the way he used to?

He said it was just the way it went when couples had been together for a while. The puppy love phase fades. But it hadn't even been a year. What would it be like in five years? Ten? I prefer to have sex every day. He suddenly did not have an interest in sex with me. He stopped complimenting me. And, frankly, that shit matters. Sex and compliments are free. Screw jewelry. Tell me I'm pretty and fuck me silly. Tell me I'm smart and kiss me till I dissociate. Tell me I'm all you could ever want and you'll never leave. I'm not complicated. At least not in that way.

Then he stopped acknowledging my little hidden love notes. I had kept up that habit since I ran out of the romance novel postcards. Now I was leaving tiny envelopes made of bright colors and old Eastern European maps that were filled with teeny-tiny cards with little messages of affection. Some were sweet:

"I will love you until I get osteoporosis!" Others were silly: "I think it's adorable when you fart in the morning and think I can't hear you."

Then one day, I caught him finding one, reading it, and sticking it in his pocket without smiling, acknowledging it, or saying anything to me.

He spotted me watching him.

"Did . . . you . . . need me to say something every time?" He looked tired.

"I—just won't do that anymore." I had to leave the room so I didn't cry in front of him.

I wasn't giving him love notes for a reaction, or a thank-you. But I did want them to make him happy. It hurt to see his utter indifference. It was embarrassing. Here I was throwing my lace-trimmed-self at him, getting rejected on the regular. He was bored, and I was leaving him love notes—like an asshole. Had I fooled myself completely, here?

Meanwhile, his little observations, annoyances with me, were growing every day. He would say, "You always . . ." and tell me something he couldn't stand about me. I told him this bothered me. I'm open to criticism, but could he please balance out the negative with the occasional compliment?

I was very clear. Because I'm a thirty-nine-year-old woman and an excellent communicator. I don't need to be a mystery. I tell a man what I want and need from him.

However, my asks went unanswered. He didn't want to change. Even though he already had, once.

Instead of getting outwardly angry, I made myself smaller. I started apologizing constantly and jumping every time he said my name, bracing myself for another criticism. I always felt he was watching me, looking for something to pick at. This must have been in my head to a certain degree, but it didn't entirely start with me. He kept telling me to calm down. He wasn't going to break up with me. I had become neurotic, needy, and jumpy. I was not the version of myself he had fallen in love with. I'm still not sure if I was being too sensitive, or if he was too critical. The truth is probably somewhere in between. The anxiety had me start picking at the skin on my legs, and soon I had little scabs dotting my thighs as a result.

The Man started frequently telling me that I was talking too loudly. It wasn't a criticism that I had ever received before, but it was another thing that made me self-conscious. I felt I was taking up too much space in the world.

Constantly on edge, I was always waiting for the next thing I did wrong to be held up to my face—often brought to my attention in a tone like one my father used when I was little. He had no idea how he sounded—and generally he wasn't malicious. But the voice he used when he was frustrated or correcting me made me shrivel up inside. Plus, I wasn't consciously thinking that the baby stuff had been a lie, so therefore everything else he said must be a lie, too—but it was there on a subconscious level. I started walling myself off. I couldn't trust him. He broke something with us.

At one point, I had two of my brothers and several friends in town, staying at the house and visiting us. In front of my friends, The Man called me over to the kitchen from the next room with a serious tone.

"Valerie, can you come here, please?" He beckoned me with one hand while keeping the other on the counter; his fingertip was white from the pressure he was applying as he pointed at a tiny dollop of sriracha that I had apparently gotten on the marble when I was putting the hot sauce on my food.

"Do you see this?" he asked, his voice sharp.

"Yes," I said, my own voice meek and my face reddening as I realized my friends and family were watching this humiliating exchange. "I must have spilled some on the counter. I can clean it up."

"This erodes the countertop and can damage the marble. You need to clean it up right away." His delivery was firm and parental.

I promised it wouldn't happen again and his body relaxed, and gradually, everyone went back to having a good time. But the moment made me feel like a scolded child.

Both of my brothers told me that The Man had "a serious Dad vibe."

This wasn't great news, given that my father had long disapproved of me and hadn't spoken to me in at least two years by this point. Was my love for this man based on some unhealthy father–daughter shit I still hadn't dealt with? Was I seeking out a man who would make me feel just as worthless and yearning for acceptance as my father had made me feel?

In other ways, on so many other days, he was wonderful. He made my fortieth birthday the best birthday of my adult life. He surprised me with decorations and a birthday cake that looked like a bottle of Jameson, and even rented a big van to take me and all my out-of-town guests on a tour of D.C. to see the capital's sights. Most importantly, he was again the doting, warm, complimentary boyfriend with whom I had fallen in love.

Yet, just like in my childhood with my father, whose moods—calm and loving or explosive and angry—I could never anticipate, I was always on guard, never completely relaxed anymore around The Man. He never raised a hand to me, and rarely raised his voice. Looking back, every criticism made me feel exactly the way my father did when he would go over my math homework. I don't even know that it's The Man's fault that I was so sensitive to his tone and delivery. But the sense of safety and home he had once brought me was replaced with a constant low-grade anxiety. I felt like someone was persistently tugging on the thread that held me together; I was unraveling.

Every day, I thought of the children I wanted to have and would go through the internal bargaining about how wrong this current reality felt for me.

The turning point came shortly after learning that I had to have surgery. It was not a major procedure, but it wasn't minor, either. The morning afterward, I was up and around and fairly chipper when The Man left at seven thirty a.m. to help his best friend with some work around the house. He texted me several times throughout the day, each time saying he had been delayed but would be on his way home soon. I didn't say anything about the fact that I had started bleeding profusely from my surgery site and was scared and in excruciating pain, because each time, I genuinely thought he was coming home. Plus, he had developed a prickliness whenever I asked him when he was coming home—as if he thought I was trying to control him. I didn't want to push him when he was already feeling that way.

Hours passed, and another couple, two neighbors, stopped by to see how I was healing from my surgery. Seeing me in obvious pain, they couldn't believe The Man had left me alone and not asked all day how I was doing. I didn't want to lie, but I was embarrassed for The Man. I didn't know how to explain his absence to them. I didn't know how to explain it to myself.

Finally, I woke up on the couch when I heard the door unlock around eleven thirty p.m. He came in, drunk and moody—which was admittedly out of character for him. I told him I was tired and that we should talk in the morning. He stumbled up the steps and went to bed while I cried myself back to sleep on the couch.

The next day he was resolute: I had been passive aggressive and should have just told him I wanted him to come home. I explained my side of the story; each time he texted me, he had said he was on his way, so I didn't think it was necessary to ask him to leave if he was already heading out the door. Eventually he went through his texts and realized I was right. His eyes got really big when I explained how I had let my incision site just pour blood in the toilet. I had to scrub the bowl with a toilet brush because the inside of the bowl was left rust-colored from all the blood, even after flushing. He said he felt bad, though he didn't actually say the words "I'm sorry."

It was all the stranger because he had taken wonderful care of me during a prior surgery that I had been through just four months earlier. He brought me fluids in bed, gave me ice packs, and made sure I ate and took my pain medicine at appropriate intervals. I knew he was capable of being supportive. In this moment he clearly didn't want to be there for me. And it hurt.

We patched things up. But I couldn't shake my uneasiness about the whole situation. A week later we sat down to talk about the challenges in our relationship. I explained I was still struggling with the fact that he was so indifferent and absent after my surgery. For context: The Man was an absolute infant when he was sick. All it would take was a bit of a runny nose and some congestion for him to throw his body at the couch and moan about the pain he was in. I, a born nurturer, would jump into action in these moments. I would massage his face to drain his lymphatic fluid, rub his neck, and bring him tea and a heating pad. I took care of this man. I never made him beg for it. Why didn't he do the same for me when I had an actual surgery?

Something had felt off in the power dynamic of this relationship since I gave up my baby plans for him and moved away from my entire support network in D.C. I could feel it in my marrow.

I was trying to find the words to explain this, and we were just talking, calmly, as we did. The Man and I didn't ever yell. We were rational.

And then he said something he wouldn't be able to come back from.

"It's so hard trying to train you," he said, holding his hand up, palm facing me, fingers spread wide. "It's like I have to shove your face in it." As he said these last words, he shook his hand in the air, miming shoving a dog's face in poo.

Astounded, I sat quietly for a moment as I thought about this. Then I said, "Do you respect me?"

He paused, thought about it. "Mostly," he said.

And that was not enough respect for me.

In those few moments, I knew it was over. I didn't want to end things. I loved him desperately. But his words had broken the spell I had been under.

What was I doing, cowering in my own home? I'm not a woman who skulks around in fear. I'm not a taker of shit. What had I become in this relationship?

The revelation washed over me, simultaneously breaking my heart and setting me free.

That night, as The Man laid snoring behind me, I got on my phone. Much to my surprise and relief, the apartment right next door to my old one—with the same massive, shared backyard—had just miraculously become available for rent. I immediately emailed and texted the building manager—I had moved out on good terms, and they loved me. I also put in an application online and texted the current tenant (my friend Rita) to ask about viewing the place. Then I looked at my finances. I had just received a little bit of a bonus from work and had put it in savings. Now it was going to help me place a deposit down on this apartment so I could get my life back.

Finally, I emailed my fertility doctor and said that I was ready to move forward with plans to transfer one of my embryos as soon as possible.

In a matter of twenty minutes, I had organized everything for my life to get exactly back on the track it had been on prior to meeting The Man. I was relieved and utterly ruined. My soul ached, even though I knew I had made the right decision. I couldn't stay with someone who viewed me like a dog he had to train.

About that. The Man later apologized and expressed profound remorse for his statements. Our breakup was a months-long process, during which we engaged in the best sex of my life and talked more openly and frankly than we had since those early days of our relationship. The Man and I would go back and forth, in limbo, for far too long. He was hard to let go of.

I DID SOMETHING HORRIBLE. I didn't tell The Man that I had found a new place to stay, or that I had all but given up on us. I was truly hoping something would shift and I could stay with him—even if it cost me my $3,800 deposit and first month's rent. He was more precious to me than money. But this was about my dignity. Beyond that, I couldn't tell him the truth because his family was coming into town in a matter of days. I dreaded the thought of breaking up with him and having to awkwardly navigate my presence around his family. I didn't want to ruin their trip or be this unpleasant wart on the entire visit. I will never forgive myself for not telling him the truth. He deserved better. At the same time, I was hoping this whole breakup wouldn't really happen. That he could undo the words he had uttered.

I wound up a nervous wreck the entire visit. In a moment I'd like to think is uncharacteristic of me, I broke down crying in front of his mother and sister at one point, because he texted me from across the room that I was talking over his family. I was so embarrassed and humiliated, and I coped with it poorly. The Man was rightfully frustrated with my public scene. I was mortified by this moment. We spoke privately and agreed to just get through his family's trip and then we would talk when they left.

A few days later we stood on the porch together, waving goodbye as they drove away. After they turned off at the end of the street, The Man looked at me and said, "You want to talk?" I nodded.

We sat on either end of the couch. I nervously wrung my hands and cleared my throat. The Man looked serious and deep in thought.

"Do you think we're compatible?" he finally asked me, calmly.

"I am having some doubts," I said.

I explained that I had struggled to be around his family, because I had serious doubts about the future of our relationship from the moment he said that he was trying to train me like a dog, along with the revelation that he didn't completely respect me.

He listened. "That was fucked up," he admitted, of the training comment.

"I love you. I am in love with you," I said. "I don't want this to end. But the way things are going, I can do this for maybe another six months to two years, max."

He nodded and looked very serious.

We talked for a little bit more before he got up and said he needed to go for a drive.

It was over.

Nine days later I moved out—with his help.

Chapter Fourteen
Unyielding Gray

MY FRIEND NIKKI, A SINGLE mother by choice from my local wannabe-mommy group, was talking to me from the driver's seat, but I couldn't focus on her words. My attempts at conversation during the ride had entirely consisted of non sequiturs. I had been staring out the window from the front passenger seat, dazed as the unfamiliar surroundings of Northwestern D.C. passed me by. It was spring, and the landscape must have been saturated in the colors of cherry blossoms and splashed with a variety of graphic, floral hues, but the world looked dull and gray from where I was sitting.

It had been fourteen months since I'd moved out of The Man's house and back to my previous life in D.C. My internal fog was thick, and I was filled with dread over what I was about to face.

"Should I drop you off, or wait?" Nikki wanted to know. She squinted at me, and I could tell she was willing to stick around as long as I needed her to.

"Um, I'll be fine. Drop off. Drop off is fine," I mustered.

Inconceivable

Nikki looked at me, her concern evident by the crease in her forehead. She put on her blinker and turned into the hospital parking lot.

"I'm going to wait. Let me know when you get checked in."

I tried to smile at her and waved at her son, who was sucking on his fingers in the backseat, before hopping out of her SUV and walking into the emergency room.

It took less than five minutes before I was triaged. A very tired-looking nurse took my temperature and blood pressure before asking me why I was there.

"I want to be admitted for inpatient psychiatric care," I said, almost whispering.

"Okay," she said, patiently. Without looking at me, she asked, "What are your symptoms?"

"I can't stop thinking about killing myself."

The nurse finally made eye contact with me. Softer this time, she said, "What's going on?"

In those early weeks after moving out of The Man's house and into my new/old place, I slowly began rebuilding my life.

I relished decorating my apartment. The Man had generously given me a bit of cash so I could get set up in my new place. He said he wanted to help because of the money I spent on moving in and then out six months apart, getting rid of many of my possessions in the process. Plus, I had bought a car to live in his rural area, which I would now need to sell. I was a little embarrassed, but grateful, because his assistance allowed me to make my place feel like a home instead of a half-empty dorm room.

I was able to replace some of the furniture I'd gotten rid of when I moved in with him, and I bought a large, bright red umbrella that I erected in the backyard so I could be shielded from the sun and rain while I worked and wrote outside. I resumed my daily walks. Most importantly, I promised myself I would never again compromise my motherhood dreams for anyone.

I went through the steps to have a single embryo transferred about two months after my breakup with The Man.

The day of the procedure, I had to show up with a full bladder to make it easier for them to see my insides when they ran the tiny catheter through my cervix and into my uterus before injecting the precious bundle of dividing cells.

After the roughly five-minute procedure, the doctor and nurses left me to lay on my back—bladder still painfully full—for about fifteen minutes. I put my hands over my womb, closed my eyes, and thought: *You and me kiddo, you and me,* before launching into my usual meditation mantra.

The next day I distinctly remember feeling a twinge in my lower abdomen. I told myself that it was my baby girl embryo implanting in my uterus. Unfortunately, I was going to have to wait to find out.

It only took five days before a faint second line appeared on a pregnancy test. I was home alone when I got the results. Triumphant joy burst into every synapse in my brain, like the Kool-Aid Man busting through a brick wall. I had done it. We had done it.

My girl was with me. I'd never experienced such profound wonder and bliss. I had been waiting my whole life for this moment. It had been two years since I started pursuing motherhood.

Irrationally optimistic—I had a genetically healthy embryo, after all—I started collecting gifts from other mothers whose kids had grown out of toys, clothes, and baby bouncers. I bought supplies to make an adorable pregnancy announcement—including a onesie that read: "Expensive as fuck but worth every penny!"

I started filling out a baby book and writing notes to my little nugget. I made a baby registry. I planned.

And then I bled.

I was just shy of six weeks pregnant when I lost my baby. I went to the bathroom and when I wiped, I saw the blood; I panicked. I immediately lay down on the couch and tried to call and text my doctor—a very kind man at my new fertility clinic. I had moved on from Dr. Patronizing.

It was a Sunday. Within twenty minutes my doctor had called me back and I was ordering an Uber to go see him. In the interim, I had passed large, scary blood clots in the toilet. I could feel the tissue as it left my body. This could not be good.

When I arrived at the clinic, they rushed me immediately from the waiting room to an exam room, where the doctor used a vaginal ultrasound to confirm that my baby—just a multicellular cluster of all my hopes and dreams—was still inside of me. So was a massive subchorionic hematoma, which is a hemorrhage in which the blood starts leaking beneath the chorion membranes that enclose the embryo in the uterus.

Unyielding Gray

My doctor told me to be on bedrest and proceed cautiously. But I could already feel it was too late. I didn't feel pregnant anymore. The bloating was gone. My breasts didn't have the pendulous heaviness that they had taken on during the few short weeks that my baby lived inside of me.

That night and the next morning I passed more blood and clots. I went back to the doctor.

"The news isn't good," he said, as he slipped the vaginal ultrasound out of my body. He and the nurse left me alone to cry.

I moaned and I screamed like an animal caught in a trap. I wailed to my mom in the Uber on my way home.

"I want to die," I screamed. I meant it.

"Oh, baby girl, I'm so sorry, I'm so sorry," she said. There was nothing else she could do.

I CALLED HIM. THE MAN. I didn't even think about it. I don't even remember dialing the number. Suddenly his voice was there, on the other line, concerned.

I choked out the words: "I lost the baby!"

"Do you need me?" he asked.

"Yes," I said, choking back tears.

He left work at eleven a.m. on a Monday to come sit with me and hold me as I cried. He rubbed my back and brushed my hair away from my face, letting me sit with my grief in silence. He didn't say anything as I zoned in and out of a fog, alternating between staring at the wall for fifteen-minute stretches and bursting into tears, or talking about how surreal everything suddenly was. It felt like someone had died. Someone had. He left later in the afternoon, once I had calmed down and another friend was on her way over to be with me. I will always be grateful to him for this kindness he showed. He was there for me, without agenda, expectation, or obligation.

I felt like a fool. I had told everyone I could think of that I was pregnant. I had been so arrogant, making these plans, envisioning a future with my baby. I loved her. Completely. I felt like I had known her spirit my entire life. I had always been waiting to meet her. Now I never would.

When people talk about miscarriages, it sounds like a single event—an extraordinarily bad day.

The thing they don't tell you is that miscarriages can take a long time. It took me eight days to lose my baby. I am grateful I didn't need medication or a D&C to end it. But losing her in slow motion was a cruelty I could not have anticipated.

Over the next few weeks, I folded into myself, wallpapering my world in black and gray as the hot ache of misery and loss coursed through my veins. For the first time (possibly in my entire life) when people asked me how I was coping, I uttered: "I don't want to talk about it."

It seemed insulting to try to find words to describe the pain and profound sense of loss. It felt like trying to move on or have another baby would be a betrayal of the child I had lost. Nothing I have written here can convey what was taken from me that day. Nothing will ever make that okay.

• • •

I FOUND SOLACE IN LISTENING to stories from other women who have been through the same hell. Helen, who had used her gay friend as a sperm donor, had the misfortune of losing her baby just as *Roe v. Wade* was overturned. A longtime Democrat and supporter of abortion rights, she was flattened by all of the discussion that ensued about how an embryo isn't really a person. She was nine weeks pregnant when she lost her baby.

After the first ultrasound, she said: "I let myself get excited, partially, because I've seen it and partially (because) I'm looking at my little app, and it's like, 'Your chance of miscarriage is four percent.' And I'm like, Okay, there's a ninety-five percent chance it takes . . . I started looking at baby announcements on Etsy. I started filling out the baby book. I started telling some close friends. I was like: This is happening."

The following Monday she started bleeding at work.

The nurse at her doctor's office wasn't helpful. She told Helen that she would know if she was miscarrying because the bleeding would get heavier. If that happened, she was instructed to go to the hospital. She begged for an ultrasound, but the nurse couldn't get her in until the following Wednesday.

In the interim, the bleeding mostly stopped, except for some occasional spotting. She started to feel hopeful that the baby could be all right. First trimester spotting is common, after all. The days passed and it was time to go in for the ultrasound.

"I went in, and they were like, 'There's no heartbeat.'"

Just forty-eight hours later, the US Supreme Court came back with the decision reversing *Roe v. Wade*.

Helen couldn't face making a decision about getting a D&C or letting the baby pass naturally. She went home and waited.

"I didn't want this pregnancy to end," she said. She thought: "You can't make me. If it happens, it happens, but I'm not helping. No, absolutely not."

In the meantime, she was stung by the discussions in the news and among friends about abortion and when a fetus becomes a human. She believed in preserving a woman's right to choose, but not at the expense of the feelings of every mother who experiences a pregnancy loss.

After a few weeks she started to make peace with things. Helen went back to the doctor and asked for the medication to help the rest of the baby pass from her womb.

The nurse "had to do an ultrasound. It was required. I also had to sign a paper saying I consented to terminating the pregnancy, which the doctor apologized for. She was like, 'I'm sorry, this is a federal regulation and I have to do it.' She's like, 'Don't even read it, just sign your name at the bottom.'"

She took the first pill before leaving the clinic. The doctors had told her that she was going to experience pain, but that she shouldn't bother going to the emergency room because they wouldn't do anything to help. So, she stopped at a dispensary (cannabis is legal in California) and asked for something that could help her with the physical pain she was about to endure. Then she went home to wait.

Helen ate some cannabis edibles—not something she made a habit of—and tried to settle in for what her body was about to go through. Within an hour she got "very, very high."

"I felt like I was waiting for my own execution," Helen said of the hours that followed. She spent some time thinking of Frida Kahlo and Catherine of Aragon, two women who had terrible fertility journeys.

Frida Kahlo had several miscarriages and at least three abortions for medical reasons; it's believed her pregnancies were terminated when it became apparent that she couldn't safely survive them due to previously being impaled in a freak bus accident. Her painting, *The Flying Bed*, depicts Kahlo in bed, with three red threads coming from her womb and connecting her to a baby hovering above the bed, a snail to the right and a model of the female reproductive system floating off to the left. It was painted following Kahlo's miscarriage in Detroit.

Catherine of Aragon, on the other hand, suffered five miscarriages or stillborn pregnancies and only produced one child—a girl—much to the disappointment of her husband, King Henry VIII, who divorced her after twenty years of marriage for her failure to produce a male heir. She died in isolation, never living to see her daughter, Mary, become the queen of England.

Helen wanted to be alone and felt some comfort from the thought of being connected to other women in history who had also known the unique pain of losing a child.

The doctors had warned her that she might pass her fetus and actually see its tiny body. Helen shuddered at the thought, but then on the first day of her medically induced miscarriage, she looked down into the toilet bowl and saw the miniature baby with its tiny hands and a few wisps of hair—and she was grateful to have evidence of the precious life that had been with her for those few short weeks.

Helen put the baby on a piece of paper. She set it on the kitchen table because at first she didn't know what to do with it.

A few hours later, she began wandering in the house and found a little box, the kind one uses to gift a piece of jewelry.

Helen was raised Greek Orthodox, and though she never goes to church these days, she found a candle and a religious icon and made a little shrine for the baby on her kitchen table.

Then she went back to bed and went in and out of a can-nabis-induced haze, during which the reality of her loss would periodically hit her in waves, coupled with an urgent need to decide what to do with the fragile little body she had sitting in the next room. She didn't want to bury it in the ground, because she rents her apartment and would eventually leave.

"I have a lime tree that's in a pot. And I buried it in the lime tree," Helen said, wiping away tears at the memory.

The act of burying her child, the ritual of her childhood religious experience—it was all part of the healing process for Helen. She gave herself time to recover from the trauma and loss. And gradually, she felt ready to return to her conception jour-ney. She's now meeting with a fertility specialist to determine the best strategy for making her a mother.

. . .

Unyielding Gray

SOMEHOW, I DIDN'T DIE. I kept breathing and waking up in the morning, and eventually found things to laugh at and make me happy. I gave myself room to envision my life without a child for the first time, because I needed to be able to look at my future reflection in the mirror and still be able to love myself.

I still had one embryo on ice, but I worried that I would miscarry again. So I had my third egg retrieval, an eight-week process that resulted in two measly eggs. Neither fertilized.

I began to accept that motherhood might not happen for me, at least not the way I thought. I gave myself time to grieve the miscarriage. Nearly a year—during which I went out with friends, danced in public, and sang karaoke. I indulged in whiskey and stopped taking eighteen supplements every morning. I let myself have fun and just be who I was before my entire life was about the question of my eventual motherhood. I did not resume smoking.

Months passed. I turned forty-one. It was time to get back on track and prepare to transfer my last embryo. It had been three years since I finally said to myself out loud that I wanted to be a mother, since I made myself a promise that it would happen. And still, all these years older, here I was with a bassinet in my bedroom operating as the most expensive laundry basket in the history of the spin cycle.

I began taking all the right steps. I talked to my doctor and found out one of the medications I used to manage my depression can interfere with lactation—and I wanted to be able to breast-feed. I stopped taking it. After about a week I felt fine, so I figured I didn't really need it after all.

At the same time, I learned that my new health insurance (I had changed jobs) wouldn't work with the same clinic that had made my embryos. Changing clinics was going to require me to shell out $1,500 just to move the embryo from one location to another clinic roughly six blocks away.

Additionally, I was required to get a new psychological screening, as was the donor, plus we would need a therapy session together—all paid for out of my own pocket, of course.

Every time I crossed one hurdle, my insurance company, clinic, or embryologist would find several more. I wanted to transfer my embryo by March. By May, I still had no idea when or if my embryo would be accepted by the new clinic. The administrative process of simply reviewing the embryo's records cost $450 and was expected to take up to three months—with no guarantee that they would "accept" my embryo.

With growing panic, I realized that my fertility, my ability to ever have a child of my own, was being held hostage by the entire system. These requirements meant to protect me were all but guaranteeing I would be forty-two before I even had my shot with the last embryo. Bizarrely, I longed for the control I had when I could just drop into a Facebook group and see the promise of a new donor, the time when I was naïve enough to believe that was the only thing I'd need to solve in my conception journey. Those days were long gone.

Every day I felt water was rising around me. I would try to plug the holes and patch the cracks with the little remaining hope I had left. I was running out of time.

And then, it was Mother's Day weekend. This was supposed to be my first one as a mom. If I hadn't lost my daughter. But I didn't lose her. I hated that we used such weak, meaningless words to describe what I was going through. She wasn't a pair of keys, or a remote control. She was my baby and she died.

I was drowning now, gasping for air. The water was coming down from overhead and up from below.

Making things worse, my mom and I had barely been talking. My father, who hadn't spoken to me in three years at this point, had retired. As a result, my mom had a hard time getting a moment away from him to talk to me—and if he knew she was speaking to me, he would pump her for information, which made me uncomfortable.

"Mom, you live in a huge house. Can't you just find a room to sneak away to for a few minutes?"

"He follows me around!" she said.

"Can't you tell him that you want to have a private conversation with your daughter?"

"Then he'll want to know what's going on with you, and you don't want that."

"Can you tell him that I've asked you not to share my personal information? You're basically enabling him to continue to not talk to me. If he's so curious about me, why hasn't he picked up a phone in three Christmases, birthdays, and every other holiday in between?"

"Well, then he's going to say I'm not allowed to talk to you."

Her words hung in the air for a single, excruciating beat.

"Mom. You're a sixty-five-year-old woman. You're going to let your husband tell you whether you can talk to your own daughter?" I tried to keep my voice calm, but hot, angry tears were pouring down my face at this point.

"You know I didn't mean it like that, Valerie. This is incredibly hard for me. I don't like being in the middle of this."

She had a point. He was her husband. And I hated seeing what this wedge between my father and me was doing to my entire family, especially my mom. I asked her to try to make more time to talk. But it felt like she was always rushing me off the phone, saying my dad would be home any minute.

And now, on Mother's Day weekend, I needed her more than ever. I sent her flowers, but only spoke to her for about two minutes on Sunday. I was sinking, and my mom was usually my go-to lifesaver. But I didn't want to burden her more with my demands when they were causing her so much stress.

And so, the unyielding gray returned, covering me in a thick cloak of ugly thoughts and enticing me with its dead-end plans. Old words, the bad words that had plagued me in my darkest days, had snuck back into my daily flow of consciousness. Intrusive words like "I want to die." I would catch myself involuntarily gazing at my wrists and visualizing them splitting open, blood spilling onto my white shag carpet. I wondered, at length, about how it would feel as my body slowly had less and less blood to sustain my heart.

My womb, a vacant, broken failure, mocked me. Each month my menses came, but to what end?

I held up a mirror to my life, and my entire existence looked like a silly facade of meaningless accomplishments on full, phony display.

The same questions echoed through my head: *What is the point of a life without children? Without legacy, someone to love, someone to mourn you, bury you?*

This was the truest death. A life absent the sounds of children laughing, and then the final curtain call of utter, permanent erasure.

I'm not sure if I decided that I needed to ask for help when I collected a box of all the things that I didn't want my family to find after I died: vibrators, mortifying old journals, and a collection of disturbingly old condoms that probably were expired anyway, among other random unmentionables.

Maybe it was all the research I was doing that made me ask for help. I had considered overdosing on pills, but I wasn't sure I had enough benzos to do the job. A little Googling led me to another conclusion: Helium. When you inhale helium, you don't exhale carbon dioxide. So, you can slowly suffocate to death without even realizing it. You just fall asleep.

I think I finally realized I needed help after I had called enough local party stores to establish that there was a helium shortage in the greater-D.C. region.

The next morning, I emailed my boss and my psychiatrist.

"I'm having a health issue. I'm not sure what's going on, but I need to go to the hospital," I wrote to my boss. Wonderful human that she is, my boss asked zero questions. She didn't know about the miscarriage. I hadn't told my work about my pregnancy efforts because I was worried about how it could affect my job security. I wouldn't be a protected class until I was pregnant.

"No problem. Take care of yourself," she wrote.

I emailed my psychiatrist, saying only: "I am having major suicidal ideation. I am not okay."

She was familiar with my background of periodic major depressive episodes—and of the miscarriage. She got back to me quickly and we spoke via video conference. I think my appearance stunned her. I joined the video call from bed, and I hadn't showered in at least five days. My psychiatrist was used to seeing me put together, with makeup on, or at least ruddy-faced and sweaty after a long walk.

She listened as I explained that I had hit a rock bottom with my mental health that was beyond anything I had experienced in at least a decade. I said that I needed help. I couldn't help myself. I couldn't make myself do life.

"I think now might be a good time to consider short-term inpatient treatment," she said. I agreed, and she emailed me links and contact information for two different facilities.

I wrote a message in the group chat with the fellow wannabe mommies (who were all mostly just mommies now) asking if anyone could give me a ride to the hospital. I had sent some worrying, despondent messages in recent days, triggering several of them to reach out and see if I was okay. So my request wasn't a surprise, but a relief.

I packed a bag and Nikki showed up, graciously, to drive me to Sibley Memorial Hospital.

I spent the night in the emergency room. They confiscated my phone "for my safety" and put me in a room with big glass windows so they could keep an eye on me. The next morning, I was admitted to the seventh floor.

I wasn't allowed to have any clothes with drawstrings, or a mirror (broken glass becomes a knife), and I eventually discovered I had to shave my legs in front of a nurse. I couldn't wear shoes, just the standard-issue socks with rubberized pads to prevent slip-and-falls.

For the moment, I was not the boss of me. This was foreign and uncomfortable, but also, I realized, necessary.

My first night in the psych ward I was in my sterile white room, rocking back and forth in the bed in an instinctive effort to self-soothe, like the Romanian orphans I had seen on the news in the nineties. I was crying quietly (or so I thought).

Eventually, a nurse came in. "Valerie, what is wrong?" she asked in her thick Caribbean accent. Her tone was stern.

"I'm sad," I said, lamely.

"Why?" she said, still stony.

"I've been going through fertility treatments for three years, and it's not working, and I'm scared. I don't see a point to a life without children."

She crossed the room, sat on the edge of my bed, and said, softly, "Me too."

I stopped crying and sat up, stunned.

"I have been trying for three years, and on Wednesday my doctor said there is no use trying any more rounds of IVF," the nurse said, now weeping herself. "I don't know what to do. I know I would be a good mother."

She wrapped her arms around me and rested her head on top of mine. I hugged her back. She smelled clean, like soap and baby powder. Her long braids draped over my head, further nestling me in her embrace.

We held each other like that and cried together, and talked about everything we'd been through and how exhausting it was pretending to be happy or "fine" all the time.

She hugged me so tightly and I didn't feel alone for that one moment. For the first time in a long time.

I went to sleep soon after, and had a deep, dreamless slumber. Eight hours of peace.

I had veered from desperation to this place of gentle comfort, because somehow, this wonderful person was sent to support me in exactly the way I needed. It was the beginning of my healing.

Over the next six days I was put back on the medication I had stopped taking two months before. My mental health was more important for any future baby than breastfeeding. I went to group art therapy and ate a lot of pudding. I had space to feel my feelings without having to live in the world and got a break from putting on a low-budget, unconvincing performance as myself, or at least the person who I actually wanted to be.

Slowly, the fog retreated enough that I got my coping skills back. And the hospital released me.

My mom arrived the day after I got out. We talked. A lot. Over the next week, she helped me reorganize my bathroom, took me grocery shopping for healthy food, and generally showed up for me in every possible way. She hadn't realized how hard the distance between us had been for me. We have been back to speaking nearly daily ever since.

Since that time, I've refocused on my friendships and my relationship with my mom and brothers. This, more than anything, led me back to a restorative place of mental and emotional health.

THREE MONTHS LATER, I decided the time had come for my final embryo transfer. I switched to another clinic (now my fourth!), because it didn't charge as many bogus fees.

"You've been through quite a lot," my new doctor said after she read my medical record. Unlike Dr. Patronizing, she didn't make me feel like a number or a dollar sign. It may have helped that she was a woman. She took an hour with me at our first appointment and reassured me that the clinic would do all they could to help.

But after spending $500 to rent a cryotank and transport my embryo from the old clinic to the new clinic, I hit a serious roadblock: my new clinic said that a major "labeling error" by the former clinic prevented them from performing my embryo transfer.

I soon learned that the issue came down to the fact that I had used a known donor. My previous clinic had labeled the sperm as coming from a known donor on one piece of paperwork, and from a sexually intimate partner on another. Yes, both were true, but in order for the new clinic to carry out the procedure, the two pieces of paperwork had to match.

"No fertility clinic in the United States would transfer this embryo, Valerie," my new doctor said to me. "We would risk losing our license and having our lab shut down. I'm so sorry, Valerie. I'm so sorry."

I received this news while I was on a walk in my neighborhood. I wasn't in a place where I could cry in despair without looking like a loon. But this time I wasn't sad—I was angry at the red tape and the fertility industry's idiotic policies. My previous clinic could transfer the embryo, but they weren't covered by my insurance, and it would cost thousands out-of-pocket for the procedure.

I sat down and wrote a lengthy email to the doctor there, explaining the situation and the egregiousness of the labeling mistake. A friend who was a lawyer advised me on the tone and content of the note—at the end of the day this was a medical error for which I shouldn't have to pay.

The doctor immediately replied and said he would research what happened. Twenty-four hours later, he called to say the clinic would do the transfer at no cost. Even better—he was prepared to expedite the timeline so I could start medication and get the process underway immediately.

I had already done much to prepare for the big day: I had lost twenty-eight pounds, attended twice-weekly acupuncture appointments, eliminated gluten and sugar from my diet, cut out alcohol, and returned to an intense supplement routine.

But my head still wasn't in the right place. In fact, my transfer date had to be pushed back twice because my uterine lining wasn't thick enough to welcome an embryo. My doctor said it was stress—he noticed my heart rate was high (unusual for me) and my hands were shaking. He instructed me to sleep and meditate more, and basically to get a grip.

He was right. I was still carrying the trauma and pain of three years of fertility struggles. It was time to make peace with the past if I was ever going to move forward.

I had some additional sessions with my therapist. I was still holding on to so much guilt about my miscarriage, but I soon realized that having this embryo transferred didn't mean that loss needed to be forgotten.

Finally, after two weeks, my lining was thick enough to safely transfer an embryo. It was time.

That day, I changed into my light blue surgical gown, put my regular clothes in a locker, and padded out to the transfer room in the rubber-bottom hospital socks that the nurse had provided. Once again, my bladder was full, my feet were in stirrups, and the doctor was inserting a long catheter through my cervix. I watched the ultrasound screen, rapt, as the catheter ran into my uterus. When the doctor injected the embryo, it created a momentary spark on the screen where it landed inside of me. Now it was time to wait.

I WAS IN NEW YORK CITY just four days later to be with my mom, who had flown in from Seattle. I dropped my suitcase in the hotel room and was walking to meet her for lunch when something came over me: I needed to buy a pregnancy test. Immediately. I stopped at a pharmacy and bought a pack of three. It was incredibly unlikely that I would get a positive test just four days after an embryo transfer, but something told me to try anyway. I figured I'd wait till later when I was back in the hotel room, so I sheepishly opened the box, stuck the tests in my purse, and continued on my way to the restaurant.

Seeing my mom is always special. Her hug smelled expensive and familiar. We sat down, started chatting, and quickly ordered a mix of small plates. We giggled and talked about our plans for the next few days in the city, and I rambled on about my hope that the transfer would work. Almost an hour into the meal, I excused myself from our discussion about baby names to use the restroom. I simply couldn't wait another moment to take a pregnancy test. Alone in the dimly lit bathroom, I plucked one from my purse and dubiously unwrapped it.

I thought: *It's going to be negative. Obviously. But at least I can stop thinking about it for today.*

I hovered over the toilet and clumsily peed on the stick. Once I finished and got my pants back on, I looked at the test. I felt dizzy, and time seemed to stop for a moment. It was indisputably positive. Regaining my equilibrium, my heart exploded and adrenaline started churning through my body. I was certain that I could hear my heartbeat. I made my way back to the table and thrust the test at my mom.

"Woah, that is definitely positive. Not even a maybe!" she said. Her eyes were full of surprise and wonder.

"Mom! I'm pregnant!" I wanted to cry. Instead, I just felt my face burning red with excitement and sat there with a stupid grin as the waiter brought the latest course to the already over-flowing table.

The rest of the weekend I levitated around the greatest city in the world, awestruck that my baby boy was with me. I could *feel* him, his spirit. I knew I wasn't alone.

It didn't take long for the excitement to give way to fear. Any woman who has had a miscarriage knows. When is it safe to believe your baby will stay with you? When is it safe to announce the good news? When is there a guarantee that everything will be okay? Unfortunately, the answer is never.

I've come to understand that is the life of a parent: worrying about your kids. That heavy, unyielding fear is a privilege that I'm embracing. Because once you get the most precious thing in the world, how can you *not* fear losing it? But I chose not to dwell too long, or too often, in the shadow of that fear.

Instead, I chose to feel gratitude as I watched my embryo grow from a small blob with a flickering heartbeat on the ultrasound screen to an actual, unmistakable baby with all the fingers on his hands wiggling, his feet kicking, and his little bum bouncing up and down inside of me.

I'm now sixteen weeks pregnant, and though it's too early to feel him move, I believe this little boy is sticking with me. I believe I'm going to be a momma. I believe I already am.

Notes

Chapter One: Chasing Babies

12 *the prior five years before this uptick, birthrates were steadily declining by roughly 1 percent a year*: Michelle J. K. Osterman, Brady E. Hamilton, Joyce A. Martin, et al., "Births: Final Data for 2021," *National Vital Statistics Reports*, vol. 72, no. 1 (Hyattsville, MD: National Center for Health Statistics, 2023), https://doi.org/10.15620/cdc:122047.

14 *In 2021, new births among women ages twenty to twenty-four declined by 3 percent, but they rose as much as 5 percent for women ages twenty-five to forty-four*: Ibid.

17 *Nearly 171,000 American women used sperm from a bank to get pregnant in 1995. By 2016 that number had risen to more than 440,000*: Rachel Arocho, Elizabeth B. Lozano, and Carolyn T. Halpern, "Estimates of Donated Sperm Use in the United States: National Survey of Family Growth 1995–2017," *Fertility and Sterility* 112, no. 4 (October 2019): 718–23, https://doi.org/10.1016/j.fertnstert.2019.05.031, PMID: 31371048, PMCID: PMC6765402.

Chapter Three: Prolific Producers

44 *a survey of donors using a website for recipients and sperm donors to connect with each other*: T. Freeman, V. Jadva, E. Tranfield, et al., "Online Sperm Donation: A Survey of the Demographic Characteristics, Motivations, Preferences and Experiences of Sperm Donors on a Connection Website," *Human Reproduction* 31, no. 9 (2016): 2082–89, https://doi.org/10.1093/humrep/dew166.

Chapter Five: Paging Dr. Patronizing

80 *he polled his medical students to determine which among them everyone believed was the most attractive*: A. T. Gregoire and Robert C. Mayer,

Notes

"The Impregnators," *Fertility and Sterility* 16, no. 1 (1965): https://doi.org/10.1016/S0015-0282(16)35476-0.

80 *Pancoast anesthetized the woman with chloroform and inseminated her with the sperm using a rubber syringe followed by a pack of gauze shoved against her cervix*: Elizabeth Yuko, "The First Artificial Insemination Was an Ethical Nightmare," *The Atlantic*, Jan. 8, 2016, https://www.theatlantic.com/health/archive/2016/01/first-artificial-insemination/423198.

81 *the student, Dr. Addison Davis Hard, revealed the truth to the AI offspring, by then an adult*: Gregoire and Mayer, "The Impregnators."

90 *After thirty-five, the likelihood rises to more than 20 percent and reaches nearly 30 percent by age forty*: Jane Menken, James Trussell, and Ulla Larsen, "Age and Infertility," *Science* 233, no. 4771 (1986): 1389–94, https://doi.org/10.1126/science.3755843. Erratum in *Science* 234, no. 4771 (1986): 413. PMID: 3755843, https://pubmed.ncbi.nlm.nih.gov/3755843.

Chapter Six: Don't Call Them Diblings

109 *46 percent of candidates wanted information on how many children would be conceived using their sperm*: Annelies Thijssen, Veerle Provoost, Eva Vandormael, et al., "Motivations and Attitudes of Candidate Sperm Donors in Belgium," *Fertility and Sterility* 108, no. 3 (2017): 539–47, https://doi.org/10.1016/j.fertnstert.2017.06.014.

109 *17 percent said they were certain they would follow through with donating without anonymity*: Bjørn Bay, Peter B. Larsen, Ulrik Schiøler Kesmodel, and Hans Jakob Ingerslev, "Danish Sperm Donors across Three Decades: Motivations and Attitudes," *Fertility and Sterility* 101, no. 1 (2014): 252–257. https://doi.org/10.1016/j.fertnstert.2013.09.013.

117 *he believed medicine should approach human reproduction with the goal of increasing the occurrence of desirable heritable characteristics*: Kara W.

Swanson, "Adultery by Doctor: Artificial Insemination, 1890–1945," *Chicago-Kent Law Review* 87, no. 2 (2012): 591, https://scholarship .kentlaw.iit.edu/cklawreview/vol87/iss2/15.

118 *Barton used her husband's sperm to produce as many as six hundred babies through her practice*: Jenny Kleeman, "The Great Sperm Heist: 'They Were Playing with People's Lives,'" *The Guardian,* Sept. 25, 2021, https://www.theguardian.com/lifeandstyle/2021 /sep/25/the-great-sperm-heist-they-were-playing-with-peoples -lives.

119 *"Fatherhood After Death Has Now Been Proven Possible"*: Alexis C. Madrigal, "The Surprising Birthplace of the First Sperm Bank," *The Atlantic,* Apr. 28, 2014, https://www.theatlantic.com/technology /archive/2014/04/how-the-first-sperm-bank-began/361288.

119 *379, or 80 percent, of the 471 respondents were, in fact, using donor sperm for AI*: Martin Curie-Cohen, Lesleigh Luttrell, and Sander Shapiro, "Current Practice of Artificial Insemination by Donor in the United States." *New England Journal of Medicine* 300, no. 11 (1979): 585–90, https://doi.org/10.1056/NEJM197903153001103, PMID: 763271.

120 *established to collect the sperm of the world's best and brightest and then spread that high-value seed to spawn geniuses across all the land, apparently*: Madrigal, "Surprising Birthplace."

121 *The American Society for Reproductive Medicine has guidelines that call for a limit of twenty-five live births per donor, per population area of 800,000*: Practice Committee of the American Society for Reproductive Medicine and the Practice Committee for the Society for Assisted Reproductive Technology, "Guidance Regarding Gamete and Embryo Donation," *Fertility and Sterility* 115, no. 6 (2021), https://doi.org/10.1016/j.fertnstert.2021. 01.045.

122 *strict limits are enforced in other countries and jurisdictions, including the UK (ten families per donor)*: "Q&A," *Human Fertilisation and Embryology Authority*, https://www.hfea.gov.uk/donation/donors/donating-your-sperm.

122 *Seattle Sperm Bank even vaguely references its consignment program on its website and in its donor agreement*: "Purchaser Semen and Storage Agreement," Seattle Sperm Bank website, https://www.seattlespermbank.com/form-pssa.

Chapter Seven: Designer Babies

141 *He achieved all his medical breakthroughs by performing surgeries on enslaved women without their consent or anesthesia*: L. L. Wall, "The Medical Ethics of Dr J. Marion Sims: A Fresh Look at the Historical Record," *Journal of Medical Ethics* 32, no. 6 (2006): 346–50, https://doi.org/10.1136/jme.2005.012559.

141 *thirty-two states established laws allowing the government to sterilize women who had been labeled insane, feebleminded, or otherwise unable to care for themselves*: Linda Villarosa, "The Long Shadow of Eugenics in America," *New York Times*, Jun. 8, 2022, https://www.nytimes.com/2022/06/08/magazine/eugenics-movement-america.html.

Chapter Eight: The Kids Are Going to Be (Mostly) Fine

156 *children without fathers are also more likely to struggle academically and score poorly on reading and mathematics; they are also more likely to drop out of school*: Edward Kruk, "The Vital Importance of Paternal Presence in Children's Lives," *Psychology Today*, May 23, 2012, http://www.psychologytoday.com/blog/co-parenting-after-divorce/201205/father-absence-father-deficit-father-hunger.

156 *overall more likely to drink alcohol and abuse drugs in adolescence, have mental health disorders, and have bleaker outcomes in terms of income, unemployment, and homelessness as adults*: Ibid.

158 *a 2022 legal analysis in the* Chicago-Kent Law Review: Yaniv Heled, Timothy Lytton, and Liza Vertinsky, "A Wrong Without a Remedy: Leaving Parents and Children with a Hollow Victory in Lawsuits Against Unscrupulous Sperm Banks," *Chicago-Kent Law Review* 96, no. 1 (2022): 115, https://scholarship.kentlaw.iit.edu/cklawreview /vol96/iss1/5.

158 *The overall good news for parents of donor-conceived children, courtesy of a study by Golombok*: Susan Golombok, Catherine Jones, Poppy Hall, et al., "A Longitudinal Study of Families Formed Through Third-Party Assisted Reproduction: Mother-Child Relationships and Child Adjustment from Infancy to Adulthood," *Developmental Psychology* 59, no. 6 (2023): 1059–73, https://psycnet.apa.org/fulltext/2023-63676-001.html.

Chapter Ten: A Hundred Fertility Heartaches

175–76 *nearly a third of US adults would struggle to cover a $400 emergency expense*: Board of Governors of the Federal Reserve System, "Report on the Economic Well-Being of U.S. Households in 2021," May 2022, https://www.federalreserve.gov/publications/files/2021 -report-economic-well-being-us-households-202205.pdf.

176 *forty-year-old women produce an average of eight eggs per IVF cycle*: R. H. Goldman, et al., "Predicting the Likelihood of Live Birth for Elective Oocyte Cryopreservation: A Counseling Tool for Physicians and Patients," *Human Reproduction* 32, no. 4 (2017): 853–59, https://doi .org/10.1093/humrep/dex008.

181 *In the 1942 decision* Skinner v. Oklahoma: Skinner v. Oklahoma, 316 U.S. 535 (1942), available at https://scholar.google.com/scholar_case ?case=8050731321644873759&q=Skinner+v.+Oklahoma,316U.S .535(1942)&hl=en&as_sdt=80006&as_vis=1.

181 *It's estimated that only 24 percent of Americans who need assisted reproductive technology get the help they need*: ESHRE Capri Workshop

Notes

Group, "Social Determinants of Human Reproduction," *Human Reproduction* 16, no. 7 (2001): 1518–26, https://academic.oup.com /humrep/article/16/7/1518/693439.

181 *More than seven million women in the US—about 12 percent of those at reproductive age—experience infertility challenges*: Centers for Disease Control and Prevention, "Key Statistics from the National Survey of Family Growth," CDC website, https://www.cdc.gov/nchs/nsfg /key_statistics/i.htm#infertilityservices (accessed Feb. 9, 2021).

181 *Close to 10 percent of men are infertile or have low fertility*: Anjani Chandra, Casey E. Copen, and Elizabeth Hervey Stephen, "Infertility and Impaired Fecundity in the United States, 1982–2010: Data from the National Survey of Family Growth (2013)," *National Health Statistics Reports,* no. 67, Aug. 14, 2013, www.cdc.gov/nchs/data/nhsr /nhsr067.pdf.

181 *Assisted Reproductive Technology (ART) is a factor in 2.1 percent of births in the United States*: Saswati Sunderam, Yujia Zhang, Amy Jewett, et al., "State-Specific Assisted Reproductive Technology Surveillance, United States: 2019 Data Brief," Division of Reproductive Health, National Center for Chronic Disease Prevention and Health Promotion, CDC, October 2021, https://www.cdc.gov/art/state -specific-surveillance/2019/index.html.

181–82 *about half of Europe's rate*: European Society of Human Reproduction and Embryology, ART fact sheet, https://www.eshre .eu/Press-Room/Resources/Fact-sheet (accessed Jun. 2, 2021).

182 *Some of the highest ART birth rates are in Denmark (6 percent), Belgium (4 percent), and Sweden (3.5 percent)*: M. S. Kupka, A. P. Ferraretti, J. de Mouzon, et al., "Assisted Reproductive Technology in Europe, 2010: Results Generated from European Registers by ESHRE," *Human Reproduction* 29, no. 10 (2014): 2099–2113, https://doi.org /10.1093/humrep/deu175.

Notes

Chapter Eleven: Congratulations, You're a Father

194 *the self-described Christian virgin became the first-ever private sperm donor to be targeted for FDA enforcement*: Amber D. Abbasi, "The Curious Case of Trent Arsenault: Questioning FDA Regulatory Authority Over Private Sperm Donation," *Annals of Health Law* 22, no. 1 (2013), https://lawecommons.luc.edu/annals/vol22/iss1/3.

194 *The California man made 328 donations to forty-six different recipients with the intent to get them pregnant*: Laird Harrison, "CA Sperm Donor at Odds with Federal Regulators," Reuters, December 20, 2011, https://www.reuters.com/article/us-ca -sperm-donor/ca-sperm-donor-at-odds-with-federal-regulators -idUSTRE7BJ2E620111220.

195 *he was in violation of federal laws and regulations governing donation of biological tissue*: Abbasi, "The Curious Case."

195 *"Under what circumstances can the government tell you not to conceive with another person?"*: Ibid.

195 *CBER asserted in that case, "The plain meaning of the words . . . do not require further explanation"*: Ibid.

198 *The April 2015 court decision stemmed from a verbal deal that Joyce Rosemary Bruce struck with Robert Preston Boardwine*: Larry O'Dell, "Virginia Court: Dad Has Rights After Turkey-Baster Pregnancy," Associated Press, April 21, 2015, https://apnews.com/4f85e23b6b8 e4bd5a80f8aff47a922b5.

209 *"My body instantly started shaking," Kris told* The 19th, *a not-for-profit news website*: Sara Luterman and Kate Sosin, "A Lesbian Mom Raised Her Son for Two Years. An Oklahoma Judge Erased That in 15 Minutes," *The 19th*, May 20, 2022, https://19thnews.org/2022 /05/oklahoma-custody-case-lgbtq-parenting-marriage-equality.

Acknowledgments

Though writing is my greatest love, it can be a lonely toil . . . which is why I must acknowledge, with love and gratitude, Abby Vaughn. Thank you for listening for so many hours as I read excerpts aloud to you over the phone. Thank you for interrupting with good questions and terrible questions in equal measure, and for being my companion when I'm deep in the words.

To the Fabulous Bauman Boys: Nothing can check my ego like you, Mark Bauman. I'm a better person because of that accountability. As I pursued this project, I frequently returned to your advice to consider my future child when being confessional. In other words: It could have been worse. Thank you for always keeping it—and me—real. And, Drew Bauman, do you remember that time I went through that really bad thing, got really depressed, and was sleeping all day, every day? And you called me every morning at nine a.m. for six weeks to get me out of bed so I had to be a person again? I'm here to write this book, in part, because of your selfless, steadfast support. Finally, Jack Bauman, being your sister cemented my desire to be a mom. Being old enough to watch you grow from infancy into a man has been a singular gift: a sneak peek into the wonder that parents must experience—the sheer magic of watching someone becoming who they actually are.

Additional gratitude must be reserved for so many more. Dena Gudaitis, I suspected we would be friends forever when

Acknowledgments

you were there for me—essentially a stranger—through my miscarriage. I was certain of that fact when you returned the next day just to sit with me in my pain. But you really proved it when you suffered through my entire rough draft. Bethany and Nick Butler, I will always be grateful for your encouragement. As I read chapters aloud, your feedback made me believe I could really do this. We are three creative soulmates who must join forces someday. Hillary Reskin, thank you for your smarts, your stellar instincts, and for believing in me and the story I wanted to tell. Joe Shaw, thank you for your steadfast friendship over the years. Amanda Ireland, dear friend and faithful reader, I will never forget your contributions and fierce support. Karanja Augustine, comrade, thank you for seeing me through this year of agonizing over my words—I owe you a drink.

To the people behind the people: Nicole Tourtelot, thank you for believing in me and this story, and for fighting to get it out into the world. Joy Fowlkes, you saw the true potential in telling this story and opened the door of opportunity to me, and I thanked you with excessive emails at odd hours. Please accept this as a (new and improved) thank-you and an apology.

To the heroes: I was a broken high school dropout with no future when I walked into your English 101 class at Tacoma Community College, Diana Marr. You saw something in me, helped me discover that I am, in fact, a writer. You changed the entire course of my life. I will repay you, emulate you, by uplifting others. Special thanks to my mentor, Michael Gormley. I'll never be able to express how grateful I am for having your guidance and wisdom over the years. I've learned so much from you— about writing and journalism, but most importantly, integrity.

To the donors: David Conrad, my love, my darling friend, you stepped up to give me the most incredible gift. I will never forget it. Eddie, I cherish our friendship and am so grateful that this bizarre subculture brought us together. To The Lawyer: You saw me as a natural mother and gave me the gift of a true chance at my dreams. Thank you.

Thank you, all.

About the Author

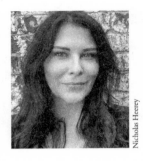

Nicholas Heerey

VALERIE BAUMAN is an award-winning journalist with nearly two decades of experience. She is currently an investigative reporter at *Newsweek*. Previously, she was a senior investigative reporter and senior legal reporter at *Bloomberg Law*, where she covered the pharmaceutical litigation beat. Bauman has also worked at *Newsday* and the Associated Press, where she covered Hurricane Katrina from the Mississippi bureau, and later the New York State legislature as a political reporter.